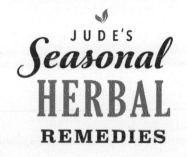

JUDE'S

Seasonal

HERBAL

REMEDIES

About the Authors

In her more than forty years of involvement with herbs, Jude Todd, CH, MH, (1942–2012) earned the titles Master Herbalist from Dominion College and Naturopathic Doctor from the American Holistic College of Nutrition. Jude was a sought-after lecturer and a frequent guest on radio shows, discussing the topic of herbal medicine.

Carly Wall, Certified Aromatherapist and author of previous titles on the subject of herbs and aromatherapy, is Jude Todd's daughter. Upon discovering the manuscript her mother was working on before she passed away, Carly compiled and edited the book to celebrate and share Jude's final work with her many readers. Carly's blog can be found at Carly's Herbal Adventures: http://www.carlys-herbal -adventures.com/.

JUDE'S
Seasonal
HERBAL
REMEDIES

Recipes for Natural Healing

JUDE TODD • CARLY WALL

Llewellyn Publications
Woodbury, Minnesota

First Edition
First Printing, 2024

Book design by Samantha Peterson and Christine Ha
Cover design by Kevin R. Brown
Interior illustrations by Llewellyn Art Department (pages 3, 4, 7, 17, 18, 21, 23, 24, 31, 32, 34, 39, 40, 43, 44, 47, 54, 57, 58, 61, 65, 66, 69, 70, 75, 76, 79, 80, 83, 89, 90, 93, 95, 100, 103, 104, 107, 108, 111, 112, 123, 124, 127, 131, 133, 134, 141, 145, 146, 149, 150, 153 & 154)

Llewellyn Publications is a registered trademark of Llewellyn Worldwide Ltd.

Information in the appendixes is taken from *Jude's Herbal Home Remedies* by Jude Todd.

Library of Congress Cataloging-in-Publication Data
Names: Todd, Jude C., author. | Wall, Carly, author.
Title: Jude's seasonal herbal remedies : recipes for natural healing / by
    Jude C. Todd, MH, ND, and Carly Wall.
Description: First edition. | Woodbury, MN : Llewellyn Worldwide Ltd, 2024.
    | Includes bibliographical references and index. | Summary: "The
    medicinal virtues of herbs and plants and the natural wisdom of our
    ancestors has been passed down to us in the time-honored traditions of
    home remedies. That tradition continues in this book through calming
    teas, restorative soaks, refreshing face creams, revitalizing shampoos,
    and so much more"-- Provided by publisher.
Identifiers: LCCN 2024012965 (print) | LCCN 2024012966 (ebook) | ISBN
    9780738776743 (paperback) | ISBN 9780738776989 (ebook)
Subjects: LCSH: Herbs--Therapeutic use. | Traditional medicine. |
    Naturopathy.
Classification: LCC RM666.H33 T64 2024 (print) | LCC RM666.H33 (ebook)
    | DDC 615.3/21—dc23/eng/20240411
LC record available at https://lccn.loc.gov/2024012965
LC ebook record available at https://lccn.loc.gov/2024012966

Llewellyn Publications
A Division of Llewellyn Worldwide Ltd.
2143 Wooddale Drive
Woodbury, MN 55125-2989
www.llewellyn.com

Printed in the United States of America

Other Books by Jude Todd

Jude's Herbal Home Remedies: Natural Health,
Beauty & Home-Care Secrets
(Llewellyn, 1992)

Other Books by Carly Wall

Flower Secrets Revealed: Using Flowers to Heal,
Beautify, and Energize Your Life
(A.R.E. Press, 1993)

Naturally Healing Herbs
(Sterling Publishing, 1996)

Setting the Mood with Aromatherapy
(Sterling Publishing, 1998)

The Little Giant Encyclopedia of Home Remedies
(Sterling Publishing, 2000)

The Scented Veil: Using Scent to Awaken the Soul
(A.R.E. Press, 2002)

For my family and special writing friends, and all who knew and loved Jude Todd.

CONTENTS

DISCLAIMER

This book is not a substitute for proper medical care. It is not intended to be a medical guide. Consult your doctor for any serious health problems. Herbs can be very potent and must be used responsibly. Some of them can be poisonous. You are responsible for your health. The publisher assumes no responsibility for the efficacy of these recipes, nor do we promise any cures. Use caution and common sense with the recipes found in this book. Many people are allergic to some plants, so do a skin patch test before using an herb in a recipe, to test for an allergic response.

SPECIAL NOTE TO THE READER

Jude Todd, my mother and author of *Jude's Herbal Home Remedies*, was working on this manuscript when she passed away in the summer of 2012. It is a collection of healing herbal recipes specially focused on what you need for each season to create natural healing products in your own home. As a healer, she was focused on what grew around her and the seasons that affected plant growth and our own bodies. She lived in Ohio, but these recipes and remedies can be used anywhere, whenever a remedy is needed. This book is a glimpse into how she lived, harvested, and preserved the precious plants, seeds, and roots for future use.

I initially found the manuscript when we were going through her things years ago and put it away in a closet. For some reason, I decided now was a good time to present it to the world. Maybe it took that much time for me to grieve properly, or maybe it is the right time to get her message out. I've done a bit of editing, added a little here and there, but essentially these are her recipes in her voice. I have been very pleased to work on this with her, even if it is in spirit.

Growing up with a mother who was interested in herbs and natural health was a blissful life that was closely tied to nature. She took her children with her into the woods to gather the roots, seeds, and leaves so she could turn them into amazing potions, lotions, or tinctures. Eventually, she went on to obtain education as a Master Herbalist at Dominion Herbal College, as well as a degree in nutrition.

My fondest memory is from the late 1960s when I was around nine years old. When she was just getting started, she decided we had to live somewhere with lots of land and wooded acres to play in. We moved to an old two-story home that had a little one-room cottage beside it. The house sat near the road on the top of a hill. Many people told us the house was haunted by an old woman, and word was she told fortunes and hid her gold coins somewhere near the giant stone fireplace that stood at the end of a large living room. My brother, sisters, and I spent hours looking for the treasure but never found it. We experienced several paranormal events, including a sighting of the old woman's spirit.

However, Mom never focused on that. This place was a dream for her. It had a beautiful yard, woods, a pond, streams, room for a large garden, and a chicken coop. She could live with the spirits if they stayed in their place. She was happy to have plenty of room to search for and grow her beloved plants. She spent her summer days canning everything she could find or grow and took organic to the next level. She began to experiment with the herbs and learned the medicinal properties and what did and didn't work.

Her first foray into herbalism was making dandelion wine. All four children were sent out to the yard with bags and told to fill them with dandelion blossoms. "Not the stems, just the flower," she said and showed us how to put two fingers under the blossom on either side of the stem and pop off the fuzzy yellow bloom head. "The one with the most in their bag gets a special treat." Of course, we all won, and the treat was a Saturday night trip to the drive-in in our pajamas.

After Mom had made her dandelion mixture, she put the bottles in the bottom of a kitchen cabinet to ferment. One night at dinner, we heard what sounded like gunshots. Terrified, everyone dove under the table and our mother burst out in laughter. "It's the wine," she said. The corks were popping off the bottles from the pressure of the fermentation process. After this, many experiments, some successful and some not, were tried. As she got comfortable with her herbal experience, she decided there was something else she wanted to try.

She decided to tackle the cottage next door. "This would make a great little store," she said as she looked around the dusty room filled with discarded furniture and debris. At this time, herbs were becoming very popular. We all spent several days cleaning the cottage. Mom sewed curtains and Dad made a checkout counter and shelving. Mom spent several weeks filling the space with organic vegetables, jellies, fresh and dried herbs, tonics, liniments, ointments, and more.

The store was only open on the weekends, but it was a wonderful little shop that did steady business. Mom loved it.

Even though we were only open on Fridays and Saturdays, inquiring customers would stop in during the week. Mom welcomed them. One weekday morning while Mom was busy canning in the kitchen, we got a knock at the door. I answered it, and there stood an elderly man in a suit and hat with round spectacles perched on his nose. He held up one of Mom's liniment jars, and it was empty.

"Can I see the healing woman?" he asked.

Healing woman. After that, that is exactly how I began to think of my mother. I often called her that too. She was so invested in helping people, and their appreciation and smiles were what she lived for. She wrote several books that contain her healing recipes.

Mom's spirit rings strong through the pages, and I know that it was her hope this book could be of some use and healing to those who study its pages. It's my hope too.

—Carly Wall

INTRODUCTION

Keeping our immune system strong is so important, and that is what healing herbs and plants are for. Herbs are not miracle workers. They in themselves do not heal you. Your physician does not heal you. Your body does all the work. By keeping our systems as chemical free as possible and making sure our bodies have all they need to build strong immune systems, we allow our bodies to do what they do best: heal. When we ingest foreign substances and chemicals through our food or medications, we allow toxins to build up in the liver and other internal organs, thus weakening our entire system.

This book gives you a wide array of herbal recipes you can create and use throughout the year. At one time, home healing was the only way to go. Early herbalists made sure their medicine cabinets had a wide variety of healing potions, lotions, and tinctures stored away. This ensured they had an answer to any problem the household encountered, no matter what time of year. This recipe book can help you stock your own medicine cabinet with simple home remedies to solve everyday problems without relying on store-bought concoctions that are often expensive and laced with chemicals.

Herbal History and Its Seasonal Connection

Ancients believed that events in the heavens reflected and affected the destinies of each and every one of us. Early wise men and women observed that the heavens do foretell the changing seasons and weather and that they guide other important events, such as plant growth. Because the history of humankind is based on agriculture, the information they learned through the years was soon used to plant and harvest crops at the best possible times and in the best possible ways according to the seasons. This practice is still observed today by farmers and gardeners. The seasons show us a circle of life that works hand in hand with nature, and by observing the seasons, we can easily follow the earth and its cycles. We soon realize that it involves everything and everyone connected to the earth.

Today we use the moon to know when the right time is to plant and harvest. Why would this not hold true for harvesting and using herbs to treat physical ills that afflict humankind?

Though there is controversy, some studies have actually shown that the full moon has some effect on our minds and health. As Leonie A. Calver, Barrie J. Stokes, and Geoffrey K. Isbister write in their article "The Dark Side of the Moon":

> The favoured belief that phases of the moon ("Luna") and extreme human behaviour are closely linked is alive and well within the health care system. This folklore, which links behavioural disturbance with the full moon (ie, the lunar phase of the brightest illumination), is not easily explained by modern science but is regularly observed. Ask any seasoned health care worker who deals directly with the more troubled public and they will argue that there is a monthly predictability of behavioural

disturbance. Those most enthusiastic about the link between disturbed behaviour and the full moon are mental health care workers, nurses in dementia units, emergency department (ED) staff and university students.[1]

Early wise men and women who practiced the healing arts learned to watch the signs of the seasons and the tendencies of strength and weakness and when they were most apt to happen. They also knew the physical was only part of the whole. The spiritual and mental state was taken into consideration along with the physical symptoms. The ones who understood the seasons and our place in the earth's cycles were the most successful healers. Because herbs are a part of the natural world, they became aware that plants were affected by the ebb and flow of the heavens. This was a new science that the healers had to become proficient in so that they could treat their patients. Ancients have long known—through trial and error—the properties of the herbs. Modern science now wants validation of that knowledge and is finding it through testing and research.

I have long held to the theory that herbs grown in a certain locale are best used to treat the people that live in that particular area because of the mineral content in the herbs. Our system is adjusted to the particular minerals of an area through the drinking water and the fruits and vegetables that grow there, and our health is dependent upon the minerals and vitamins found in herbs and other plants. The early shamans and doctors knew how important diet was to treatment and acted accordingly. Your own treatment

....
1. Calver, Stokes, and Isbister, "The Dark Side of the Moon."

might include eating vegetables and fruits native to the area. Eating healthy foods helps to prevent disease and keep blood pressure and cholesterol normal. Historically, Indigenous people lived in close harmony with nature and knew that health is dependent on what we eat, which relates to how we treat Mother Earth. We will only get back from our soil what we put into it. We must realize the wisdom of the past is of value to us and learn more about natural methods of gardening so that we work *with* Mother Nature and do not just take from her. All of life is a circle, and we must learn this if we are to survive.

I do want to caution you that herbs alone won't heal you. You must strengthen your immune system by using the herbs as you learn new and healthy ways to treat your body naturally. Herbal home remedies are not meant to replace your doctor. There are many illnesses that are best left to the experts. We are simply leading healthier lives by learning to use natural products as a way to prevent illnesses and to treat simple ills that we are all prone to now and then.

With those steps, we begin to take responsibility of our own health. We should all have a little knowledge about what a strong body means for each of us, and the seasons can more or less be a helpful road map for us to follow. We tend to have various ailments linked to the season and the time of the year we were born. If we know what to look for, and what problems might arise at a particular time of year, we can practice a preventive lifestyle. By being aware of the tendency of our health problems, we can eat a more wholesome diet that will enhance our bodies and prevent illnesses. Perhaps we can benefit by using a particular tonic if our bodies tend to show weaknesses during a specific time of year. Many herbs can be used in tea remedies. Tea remedies are an easy way to treat a person with a particular weakness during a specific season. There are many ways to practice preventive health and learn that the flow of seasons, herbs, and our health go hand in hand.

Knowledge about the use of herbs was once the exclusive domain of the shamans and healers of the temples. Now we are able to put that practical knowledge to use in our daily lives.

I consider all fruits, vegetables, trees, shrubs, and flowers to be herbs, and all herbs have their uses in ways physical, mental, and spiritual.

Healing with Flower Essences

Even flowers have healing abilities. Many people have found a spiritual aspect of healing through flower essences. It has proven to be a very interesting aspect of healing, and the process of preparing essences will be discussed later on.

The use of flower remedies first became popular through the experiments of Dr. Edward Bach. He became interested in the link between a patient's attitude, temperament, and illness. He believed that if a patient's negative attitude could be overcome, their body would respond accordingly. After talking with each patient, he knew immediately what treatment to use with that particular patient. Realizing he was treating the person for only physical problems and not getting to the root of the illness, he retired to the countryside and developed his flower remedies. Others have learned from his example and have experimented with flower essences. You can learn to make your own remedies and treat simple illnesses by using this method too.

Herbs That Grow around Us

Different plants can be found all around the world. Some of these plants are actually the same plant. They just go by different names. Other herbs may seem like they are of a totally different species, but in fact they are of the same. Even though there may be some differences, they basically have the same ingredients and can often be interchanged with one another. It is always best to use the version of a plant that grows near you, as it will have the mineral content common to your area. For example, American spikenard root (*Aralia racemosa*) is native to the Eastern United States and is often used in teas, tonics, and poultices for rheumatism and eczema. It comes from the ginseng family and has similar effects to ginseng root.

Another example. Let us say a recipe calls for valerian (*Valeriana officinalis*), which is a strong sedative. (Valerian can have adverse effects on the stomach and heart, so seek medical advice before ingesting it.) There are several different herbs that you could use to get the same effect. You could use valerian, of course, but you could also use garden heliotrope (*Heliotropium arborescens*) or Jacob's ladder (*Polemonium caeruleum*), which is also called Greek valerian. Almost all the old remedy books list Jacob's ladder in their recipes because it is widely available. If you are familiar with any of the old herbal remedy books, you know they all contained plants indigenous to the particular area the author lived in. Healers didn't have the convenience of a health food store and could not send for herbs. They gathered what they could find and used them.

Many of us are not in the position to go foraging for wild plants and herbs, and I do not advocate digging up or taking plants from the wild. Many plants are on the endangered list, and we must help preserve Mother Nature. But we can research what plants grow naturally in our area and propagate with seed or starters so we can grow our own. We can grow plants on our own land, deck, patio, or

windowsill. We then become knowledge-
able about the particular herb through
the process of planting and tending it from
babyhood to full-grown plant. We can study
its uses, and the plant will become a loved and
familiar family member.

It may surprise you to learn that you don't need a large
variety of herbs. Each herb can have different uses, and you only
need to grow a few to create many different remedies. Add herbs
slowly to your gardening project and become familiar with each one
as you go. Don't try any plant you are not completely familiar with.
Learn all you can about the herb and the properties of that plant
before attempting any home remedies. Start with three or four plants
to grow and learn about, and then expand as you go.

You may have to try different herbs to find the one that works
for you because each of us has different physical needs. A remedy
that works for a friend may not work for you thanks to your difference in body chemistry. Several tonics and recipes are listed for each
of the seasons, and one is bound to suit your needs. The easiest way
to ingest remedies is through tinctures. They are easy to prepare,
store, and use. Read through all the seasonal sections of the book
to find the easiest way to prepare and use the treatment that is most
helpful to you.

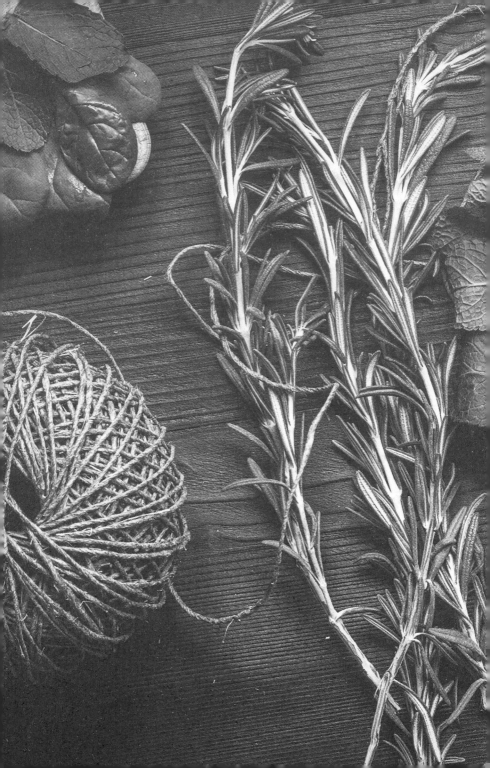

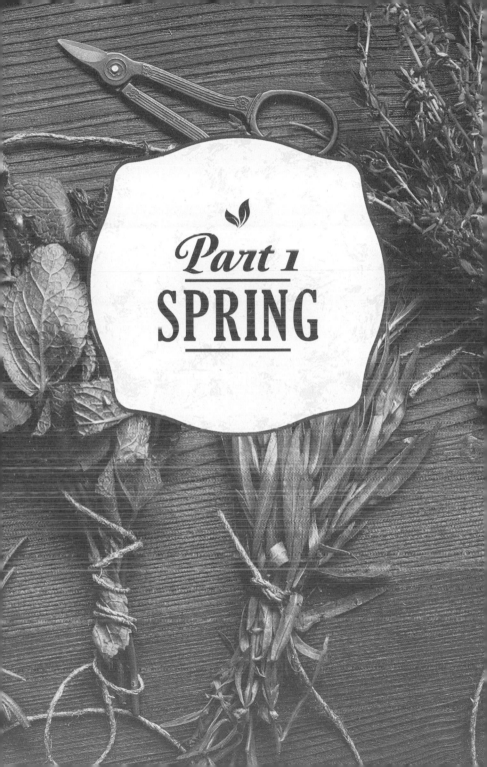

Part 1
SPRING

ONE
Early Spring
MARCH

At the first blush of spring, we see a renewal. Trees begin to bud out. Seedlings push their way to the surface where they can catch the sun's rays. The birds sing, and our spirit soars. We follow the earth in a renewal, in an awakening from winter's slumber. As we awaken, we find a need for energy and help with stress headaches. We have a tendency to have toothaches, earaches, sinus infections, neuralgia—all problems of the scalp and facial area—at this time. Emotional traumas seem to surface more easily in the spring after being dormant for the winter. Because of this, many herbs used in early spring are sedatives. With the excitement of this awakening, we have to learn to slow down and not wear ourselves out too quickly.

Herbs for Early Spring

Here are plants that I've categorized as healing herbs for early spring:

bee balm (*Monarda didyma*)
chamomile (*Anthemis nobilis, Matricaria chamomilla*)
feverfew (*Chrysanthemum parthenium*)

honeysuckle (*Diervilla lonicera*)

hops (*Humulus lupulus*)

lavender (*Lavandula angustifolia*)

lettuce (*Lactuca sativa*)

mullein (*Verbascum thapsus*)

nettle (*Urtica dioica*)

passionflower (*Passiflora incarnata*)

pennyroyal (*Mentha pulegium*)

peppermint (*Mentha piperita*)

rosemary (*Rosmarinus officinalis*)

sage (*Salvia officinalis*); do not use if pregnant or breastfeeding.

skullcap (*Scutellaria lateriflora*); do not use if pregnant or breastfeeding.

sweet woodruff (*Galium odoratum*)

valerian (*Valeriana officinalis*); avoid if you have stomach or heart issues.

violet (*Viola odorata*)

Flower Remedies

Flowers are so much a part of spring, and flower remedies are great to experiment with as the earth begins its awakening. The easiest way to prepare flower remedies is to place your choice of flowers in a thin glass bowl and cover with spring water. Allow the flowers to steep in the full sun for about three hours. This process releases the healing essences into the water. Strain out the flowers and fill vials or bottles half full with the flower essence water. Finish filling the vials or bottles with brandy or vinegar to preserve the flower essence water. Keep the water in a cool, dark area. If you are inclined, herbs can be made into a healing essence in the same manner.

The dosage is one to several dropperfuls added to water, juice, or tea. Instead of using flower remedies for physical healing, use them for their spiritual healing essences, mainly to help with emotional problems. In a way, this is a more homeopathic approach. Those who have experimented with flower essences, such as Dr. Bach, believed illness is created by a particular emotional reaction and that by treating the temperament or emotional outlook of the patient, the physical illness would dissipate on its own.

There are about thirty-eight different Bach remedies, and each are made in the same manner. You can find more information about Bach flower remedies at this website: https://www.bachremedies .com/en-us/.

Another excellent source if you are looking to purchase flower remedies is the Flower Essence Services, which is part of the Flower Essence Society, an educational and research organization: https:// www.fesflowers.com.

Here are a few flower remedies and their uses that have been quite helpful in my life:

agrimony (*Agrimonia eupatoria*): for those who hide their worries

aloe vera (*Aloe barbadensis Miller*): helps relieve feelings of burnout

angelica (*Angelica archangelica*): gives a feeling of protection so you can receive guidance from spiritual beings

arnica (*Arnica mollis*): used for treatment of deep shock or disappointment; do not ingest, only apply on the skin's surface.

basil (*Ocimum basilicum*): helps to polarize and balance sexuality and spirituality blackberry (*Rubus* spp.): helps to translate ideas and goals into workable activity

black cohosh (*Cimicifuga racemosa*): gives courage to confront abusive situations

borage (*Borago officinalis*): builds self-confidence

calendula (*Calendula officinalis*): helps put warmth in conversation and in dealing with others on a social basis

cayenne (*Capsicum annuum*): helps you accept changes and move toward a specific goal

chamomile (*Anthemis nobilis, Matricaria chamomilla*): gives a serene disposition

cherry (*Prunus avium*): helps those who have a temper to stay calm

chicory (*Cichorium intybus*): used for those who feel the need to put others right or who are too possessive

dandelion (*Taraxacum officinale*): gives energy and balances inner forces

dill (*Anethum graveolens*): helps you appreciate and enjoy all the gifts of life

echinacea (*Echinacea angustifolia*): helps feelings that have been shattered by trauma

evening primrose (*Oenothera elata* ssp. *hookeri*): helps form committed relationships

garlic (*Allium sativum*): gives a sense of wholeness

goldenrod (*Solidago canadensis*): helps balance inner sense of self with social consciousness

golden yarrow (*Achillea clypeolata*): helps to heal tendency to withdraw from social contact lavender (*Lavandula angustifolia*): gives spiritual awareness and sensitivity

mallow (*Malva sylvestris*): allows you to reach out to others

monkey flower (*Mimulus alatus*): for those fearing to be alone or with fear of illnesses or any other misfortune that could arise in the future

mugwort (*Artemisia douglasiana*): allows you to harmonize physical forces; do not use if you are pregnant.

mullein (*Verbascum thapsus*): gives a sense of conscience and truthfulness

nasturtium (*Tropaeolum majus*): gives a radiant warmth you will be able to impart to others

pennyroyal (*Mentha pulegium*): gives clarity of thought; the oil is highly toxic, so do not ingest.

peppermint (*Mentha piperita*): stops mental lethargy and helps balance metabolism

pink yarrow (*Achillea millefolium rubra*): gives loving awareness of others

Queen Anne's lace (*Daucus carota*): for spiritual insight

red clover (*Trifolium pratense*): helps you become more self-aware and contained

rosemary (*Rosmarinus officinalis*): helps forgetfulness and corrects poor connection of soul and spirit with the physical body

scotch broom (*Cytisus scoparius*): makes you feel optimistic

self-heal (*Prunella vulgaris*): causes healing from within and a sense of wholeness

St. John's wort (*Hypericum perforatum*): gives illuminated consciousness and strength to deal with bad dreams and psychic experiences

sunflower (*Helianthus annuus*): gives balanced sense of individuality

tansy (*Tanacetum vulgare*): helps you become purposeful in action toward goals

trumpet vine (*Campsis × tagliabuana*): gives freedom to express yourself verbally; do not ingest due to its high toxicity.

violet (*Viola odorata*): elevates spiritual perspective and makes you highly perceptive

yarrow (*Achillea millefolium*): creates beneficial healing forces and helps you have compassionate awareness of others

yerba santa (*Eriodictyon californicum*): frees your emotions

Relaxing Remedies

In the spring, we can often feel pressured to go in a dozen different directions after being cooped up all winter. The season of spring can especially affect the head and neck area, as well as our moods and spiritual outlooks. Though these ailments can crop up anytime, this is often the season where it will be most bothersome. Here are some of the herbal remedies you will want to have on hand to help you relax.

Tension-Relieving Tea

Nerves can cause skin eruptions. Sedative teas can be taken daily to help remedy this. Rosemary, lavender, passionflower, sweet woodruff, skullcap, pennyroyal, valerian, chamomile, lettuce, violet, bee balm, and honeysuckle tea are all good sedatives. Simply add 1 tablespoon of any of the herbs or a mixture to 1 cup of boiling water.

Cover and let steep 10 minutes. Strain and sweeten with apple powder or honey. Drink as needed to calm the nerves. Experiment with different herbs and mixtures to find your favorite.

Mental Fatigue Tea

Mix together ½ teaspoon each of sage, rosemary, peppermint, and hops. Pour 2 cups of boiling water over the herb mixture, cover, and allow to steep for 10 minutes. Strain and add a pinch of ground ginger. Sweeten to taste with honey or sugar and drink warm.

Nervous Headache Tea

Chop 1 tablespoon of violet leaves and flowers. Pour 1 cup boiling water over the herbs, cover, and steep 10 minutes. Strain and sweeten with honey. Drink ½ hour before bedtime for restful sleep.

Nervous Tension Tea

Chop ½ cup of skullcap leaves and flowers and add to 2 cups of boiling water. Cover and steep 15 minutes. Strain and sweeten with honey to taste. Drink several times a day.

Relaxant Tea

While unusual, lettuce tea is a fast-acting relaxant. Many people have lettuce available in their home; it is often on hand. Chop 1 cup of lettuce until fine. Pour 1 cup boiling water over the chopped lettuce, cover, and steep 30 minutes. Strain and drink when needed for restlessness, for fever, or simply to relax.

Headache Tea

Chop 1 cup of peppermint and pour 2 cups boiling water over the herb. Cover and steep for 5 minutes. Strain and sweeten. Add lemon juice if desired. Drink this tea at the first sign of a headache to release tension.

Mild Sedative Tea

Pour 1 pint boiling water over 1 teaspoon of dried catnip. Cover and steep until cool. Strain and sweeten with honey. Drink 2 tablespoons to help relax. Catnip is safe in small amounts, so use sparingly.

Tension Headache Bath

Place 1 ounce each of chamomile, peppermint, and lavender flowers in 1 pint of boiling water. Simmer for 20 minutes. Strain and add to your bathwater for a comforting tension-relieving bath.

Lavender Tea

Lavender is the best relaxant. This herb is extremely good for easing stress. Add 1 teaspoon dried lavender flowers or leaves to 1 cup boiling water. Cover and steep 10–15 minutes. Strain and sweeten if desired.

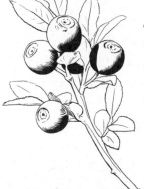

Sage Tea

Sage is an herb that helps calm someone who is agitated. Pour 1 cup of boiling water over 1 teaspoon of sage. Cover and steep 15 minutes. Strain and sweeten with honey. This tea is fast-acting to bring quick relief. Do not use if you are pregnant or breastfeeding.

All-Purpose Tea

This tea treats several different ailments. It can help you relax, relieve tension, and settle a nervous stomach quickly. It also relieves heartburn and indigestion brought on by a nervous condition. Mix together 1 tablespoon each of dried peppermint and bruised fennel seeds. Store in a tightly closed container. Place 1 teaspoon of the mix in a cup and pour 1 cup boiling water over it. Cover and steep for 15 minutes. Strain and sweeten with honey.

Skullcap Headache Tea

Skullcap is very good to treat nervous headaches. Mix together ½ cup each of dried skullcap, peppermint, and sage and place in a tightly closed container. Dosage is 1 cup of boiling water poured over 1 teaspoon of the skullcap mixture. Cover and steep for 10–15 minutes. Strain and sweeten with honey. Drink before bedtime for a relaxing sleep. Do not use if you are pregnant or breastfeeding.

Sedative Tincture

Place 1½ ounces of chamomile and 1½ teaspoons powdered peppermint in ½ quart of vodka. Steep in a warm, sunny area, shaking it daily, for 2 weeks. Strain and bottle. Dosage is ½ a dropperful under the tongue as needed. Use as a sedative for adults.

Sedative Tea

Mix together 1 tablespoon each of hops, bee balm, peppermint, chamomile, and crushed fennel seeds. Store in a tightly closed container. Add 1 tablespoon of the mixture to 1 cup of boiling water. Cover and steep for 10 minutes. Strain and sweeten to taste.

Relaxing Hops Tea

Hops are a natural relaxant. Pour 1 quart of boiling water over 1½ teaspoons of dried hops flowers. Cover and steep 10 minutes. Strain and sweeten to taste. Lemon juice may be added for taste.

Sweet Woodruff Tea

Sweet woodruff has long been used as a tonic for the heart and liver. It also has a great calming effect. Add 1 teaspoon sweet woodruff to 1 cup boiling water. Cover and steep for 15 minutes. Strain and sweeten.

Sinus Remedies

Sinus problems are common ailments in early spring—or any time of year. There are several natural treatments that can be used to help alleviate the symptoms.

Stuffy Nose Treatment

Mix 2 cups of very cold water with 1 tablespoon Epsom salts and 2 teaspoons baking soda. Dip a washcloth in the liquid and place it over your sinus area for quick relief of a stuffy nose. Repeat to keep the area cold.

Sinus Rinse

This is a saline sinus rinse with the addition of healing herbs. Use ½ teaspoon salt to ½ cup warm distilled water. Add 15–20 drops of chamomile tincture or strong tea. Make sure it is well strained before adding to the salt mixture. Place a small amount in the palm of your clean hand. Hold one nostril closed and gently sniff the mixture into your open nostril and let it drain to your throat. Repeat with the other nostril. Do this once a day until you have sinus relief.

Steam Sinus Treatment

Add ½ ounce of mullein and 1 tablespoon balm of Gilead to a kettle of water. Bring to a boil and inhale the steam. This cleans sinus passages. Do not use if you are pregnant or breastfeeding.

Vitamin C Sinus Treatment

One of the better ways to treat sinus problems is to dissolve a 1,500 mg vitamin C tablet in ½ cup of warm water. Using a dropper, apply ½ a dropperful to both nasal passages twice daily. It may sting a little at first, but it is an effective remedy.

Ear Remedy

Ear problems can also appear at this time of the year. There are many reasons for earaches, and you should be sure the earache is not caused by a medical condition best treated or prevented by your physician. Your doctor can determine this.

Mullein Earache Drops

Mullein tincture is a great herbal remedy to use for an occasional earache. To make, add a small handful of mullein flowers to a pint jar with olive oil. Cover the jar and place it in the sun for about 2 weeks. Shake the jar of oil occasionally. Strain and stir in 1 teaspoon of honey to the tincture. Honey is a great preservative and has wonderful healing properties. Use the tincture by putting a few drops in the affected ear. Put a cotton ball in the ear to hold the oil in place. Cover the ear with a warm cloth. Put a heating pad on the lowest setting, wrap it in a towel, and place it over the warm cloth covering the ear for 20 minutes. Leave the cotton ball in the ear until the pain has subsided.

Scalp and Hair Remedies

A good way to start the early spring is to use natural beauty products to slough off the winter. Since our skin is our first defense against invading organisms and chemicals, it is a good way to renew. The skin absorbs whatever we put on it, and we don't want to absorb any more chemicals than what we are already exposed to daily. There are several different natural shampoos that I've used and recommend.

Aloe Vera Shampoo

Break open a leaf or two of aloe, spread the gel on the hair, and work it in well. Wet the hair and it will lather slightly. Rinse well. The hair will have a natural sheen and be wonderfully soft. A friend introduced me to this shampoo. It promotes hair growth as well as prevents dandruff.

Rosemary Nettle Shampoo

Place a small handful of soapwort in a small stainless steel pan and pour 1½ cups of water over it. Bring to a boil. Lower the heat and simmer for 10 minutes. Remove from heat, cover, and steep until cool. Strain the liquid into a bottle that closes tightly. Place 1½ tablespoons chopped fresh rosemary and a small handful of chopped fresh nettle leaves into an earthenware bowl. Pour 1 cup of boiling water over the herbs. Steep until cool. Strain and add to the soapwort mixture. Shake the mixture well before using. Keep in the refrigerator up to 2 weeks.

Chamomile Shampoo

Pour 4 cups boiling water over 5 tablespoons of chamomile flowers. Cover and steep 30 minutes. Strain and add 4 ounces of castile soap flakes. This recipe makes about 1 quart of shampoo that is very good for the hair and scalp.

Natural Hair-Setting Lotion

No need to apply chemical preparations to your hair when you can make your own natural products. Place 2 tablespoons of flaxseeds in 1 cup of water and simmer until thickened. Strain and use as a setting gel. Quince seed works just as well; prepare in the same way. Keep the gel refrigerated. It will keep for 1–2 weeks.

Skin Remedies

Old winter can play havoc with our complexion and skin. As the earth awakens, we can awaken too by paying attention to our skin with a good diet and plenty of rest and by giving the body attention and the things it needs. This is a good time to concentrate on spiritual and physical renewal. Spend a special weekend thinking about any changes you need to make. Try it this weekend. What do you like? What do you hate? What isn't working any longer? This is a time to slow down, focus on what is needed, and appreciate what you have been blessed with. Seek new ways to express any of your artistic abilities. You may well discover a whole new calling in your life. Your lifestyle may change to one better suited to your temperament and needs, and you will become the happy, healthy individual you were meant to be. The following are skin care recipes that you may enjoy making and using anytime but especially early spring.

Violet Crème

Vitamin A is important to the body. It helps keep the skin and mucous membranes healthy, and it also helps protect against infection. Susun Weed, a renowned herbalist and women's health expert, in her book *Healing Wise*, extols the virtues of sweet violets, revealing their remarkable nutritional content. One hundred grams of sweet violet leaves provide an impressive 20,000 international units of vitamin A as well as a high content of vitamin C and other minerals.[2]

To make a crème from the herb, place 1 cup of violet leaves and flowers in a stainless steel pan. Cover the herb with almond oil and place the pan on the stove on the lowest heat setting for 10 minutes. Strain out the flowers and place the oil back in the pan. Puncture several vitamin E capsules and pour the oil into the violet mixture to preserve it. Add melted beeswax and stir until the mixture is the thickness of a face cream. You can test the thickness of the crème by taking 1 tablespoon of the mixture and placing it in the refrigerator until cooled. If it is too thick and won't spread across your skin, add more almond oil and heat to thin it. A thinner crème can be used as a lotion, and a thicker crème can be used on lips, on chapped hands, or under the eyes.

....
2. Weed, *Healing Wise*.

Sweet Woodruff Ointment

This ointment is used to treat abrasions, cuts, and other skin problems. Acne, skin eruptions, and psoriasis all react favorably to this treatment. Fill a pint jar with sweet woodruff and cover with olive oil. Place the jar in a sunny window and steep for 2 weeks. Strain and add the oil of 2 vitamin A capsules and several teaspoons of honey to the mixture. Shake well before use.

Gum and Tooth Remedies

Gum and tooth problems can arise at any time, but early spring is a good time to assess your oral health. A physician or dentist must determine the cause of gum disease. Bleeding gums are a sign of severe medical problems. For treating minor gum issues and toothaches, there are several treatments you can try.

Toothache Poultice

Mix together 2 tablespoons of sassafras root and 1 tablespoon each of hops and catnip. Store in a tightly closed container. Place 1 teaspoon of the mixture in a small square of muslin cloth and dip it in very hot water. Apply the poultice to the affected area. Repeat every 30 minutes as required for pain. Make sure you use the sassafras root only. The oil is highly toxic.

Valerian Toothache Relief

Another way to ease toothache pain is to use valerian. Make a tincture by placing the root or powder into a pint jar. Pour ¼ cup vodka (or vinegar or glycerin) over the herb, adding more if needed to cover the herb, and steep in a sunny window for 2 weeks. Strain into a small dark bottle with a dropper. Because alcohol is a preservative, the mix will last for many years. Vinegar and glycerin are also preservatives, but if those are used, the remedy should only be stored for up to 1 year. Dosage is to add several dropperfuls to a little water and drink. This can relax you so much it may put you to sleep. When you awaken, the toothache should be gone. High doses of valerian can be toxic, so take caution when using.

Willow Tea Pain Relief

Willow is a good pain reliever. Place the leaves, twigs, or bark from a willow into 1 cup of boiling water. Steep until color appears in the water. Add other herbs to flavor if desired. Soak a cloth in the tea and place over the affected tooth, or hold some tea in the mouth to speed results.

Inflamed Gum Treatment

Papaya juice heals the tissue of the gums, so if you have an injury or raw spots from dentures, you can heal the mouth fast with papaya juice. Simply take a sip of the juice and hold it in the mouth as long as possible before spitting it out.

TWO
Mid-Spring
APRIL

Early spring quickly melds into middle spring. The earth settles in to grow and bloom. Each day reveals something new and exciting. Since we are so connected to the earth, we find ourselves awakening to the call of the sunshine. During this time, we often have throat and neck issues. Preventive health care is good for this time. The immune system often needs a boost from winter's sleep. That's why tonics and blood cleansers are promoted during this season. The remedies we concentrate on here are those that purify the blood, along with treatments for sore throats, tonsils, goiters, and chest complaints. We have the tendency to be overindulgent in matters of emotional content this time of year. The herbs listed here are to relax, keep calm, and maintain equilibrium needed for decisions that should not be made while under emotional duress.

Herbs for Mid-Spring

Here are plants that I've categorized as healing mid-spring herbs:

apple (*Pyrus malus*)

coltsfoot (*Tussilago farfara*); avoid if you have liver issues.

goldenrod (*Solidago*)

horehound (*Marrubium vulgare*)

Irish moss (*Chondrus crispus, Gigartina mamillosa*)

lemon balm (*Melissa officinalis*)

mullein (*Verbascum thapsus*)

passionflower (*Passiflora incarnata*)

peppermint (*Mentha piperita*)

plantain (*Plantago major*)

sage (*Salvia officinalis*); do not use if pregnant or breastfeeding.

skullcap (*Scutellaria lateriflora*); do not use if pregnant or breastfeeding.

slippery elm (*Ulmus rubra*)

valerian (*Valeriana officinalis*); avoid if you have stomach or heart issues.

violet (*Viola odorata*)

Cleansing Tonics

Tonics take time to work on the system, so you need to use them over a period of time to give the system time to adjust and make good use of them. The herbs build up the organs that are affected by digestion, and this helps the system to use all the vitamins and minerals you ingest when you supply it with healthy, wholesome foods. Remember that herbs are not miracle workers. They simply help the system to become strong enough to take care of itself.

Here are a few tonics that can help to cleanse the blood as well as keep the sweat glands open. This allows the glands to secrete the excess poisons that may build up over the winter through self-indulgence and eating the wrong foods.

Apple Tonic

Because apple pectin is the best blood purifier, it is the herb of choice in this season of renewal. Make sure you prepare ahead and preserve some each summer and fall so you will have it on hand. It rids the system of excess water. Apple pectin can be taken on a daily basis with no ill effects. You can use it as a sugar substitute in foods and drinks to ensure you receive it daily. One way to ensure the purity of the pectin is to make your own.

Apple Pectin and Sweetener

You can make your own pectin. Simply core some apples, leaving the skin on, and thinly slice them. Place the apple slices in an oven at the lowest temperature to dry. It may take some time, but make sure the slices stay in the oven until brittle.

To make a natural sweetener, place in a food processor and pulse until powdered. Use this as a sugar substitute. This is the best blood purifier I know of, and it's a way to cut back on using processed sugar. This type of sugar does not speed up your system like cane sugar or corn syrup.

Apple Tea for Colds

Apple tea is an old Irish remedy to purify the blood, and this tea can be used for everything from colds to just plain delight. Dry apple slices in the oven and remove before they become brittle. Place 2–4 slices in 1 cup of boiling water, cover, and steep for 10 minutes. Store remaining slices in an airtight container. Remove the apple slices and sweeten with honey if desired. If used as a treatment for colds, it removes the toxins from the system quickly because it is a wonderful diuretic. It adds vitamin C to your system, and a cup daily really does seem to keep the doctor away.

Kidney Treatment Tea

Plantain makes a pleasant tea. It is a great diuretic and can quickly remove toxins from the system. Many use plantain tea to treat kidney and bladder ailments. Gather several leaves of plantain, bruise them, and place them in a cup. Pour 1 cup boiling water over the herb, cover, and steep for 10–15 minutes. Strain and sweeten if desired. Avoid high doses.

Corn Silk Tea

Corn silk is the best diuretic I know of and is great to help clean the system when overindulgence is a problem. It cleans the kidneys bladder, and removes toxins from the system. Make a tea using 1 tablespoon of dried corn silk to 1 cup of boiling water. Cover and steep about 10–15 minutes. Strain and drink. No sweetener is needed. It tastes exactly as it smells and is a pleasant tea if you enjoy corn.

Violet Tea

Violets are a great way to add vitamin A to your diet, which is good for your heart and eyes. Make violet tea using 1 tablespoon of the leaves and flowers to 1 cup of boiling water. Cover, steep for 10–15 minutes, and strain. Sweeten if desired. This tea also acts as a mild sedative and is helpful to anyone who feels overwhelmed with all there is to do in spring. You can also add the leaves and flowers to salads.

Sore Throat Treatments

Sore throats can be symptoms of serious illness. It is important to see your physician to find the root cause. Natural remedies can be used for minor sore throats.

Slippery Elm Treatment

Slippery elm is a must for sore throats caused by inflammation of the tonsils, pharynx, or larynx. The patient should drink plenty of fluids and be kept warm and comfortable during any treatment. Make a paste using 1 tablespoon of slippery elm powder and enough water to reach the right consistency. Bring 1 pint of water to a boil and add ½ cup of honey. Slowly add the slippery elm paste to the boiling water, stirring constantly until it thickens. Pour this into a sterile container and take 1 tablespoon as needed for sore throat. Store in the refrigerator 8–10 days.

Sage Sore Throat Treatment

Sage is a wonderful herb with many uses. A gargle made from sage tea is great for sore throats. Pour 1 pint boiling water over 1 ounce of dried sage. Add 1 teaspoon cayenne pepper and mix well. Steep overnight, and use as a gargle to treat a sore throat. Do not use if pregnant or breastfeeding.

Inflamed Tonsil Treatment

Sage tea can also be used to treat inflamed tonsils. Place a large handful of fresh sage in 1 pint of boiling water. Simmer until the sage is soft. Take off the heat and let the liquid cool just a bit until you can safely dip a cloth into the tea. Put the sage in the cloth, fold it up, and wrap it around the throat. Dip another cloth in the tea and wrap it around the throat as well. Keep replacing the outer cloth to keep the inner cloth warm. Make another sage tea mixture to drink during this treatment to receive double benefits. The swelling and inflammation should subside within hours. Do not use if pregnant or breastfeeding.

Beet Sore Throat Remedy

Gargle with beet juice to treat a sore throat. This will greatly ease any throat pain.

Thyme Sore Throat Gargle

Thyme is antiseptic in nature and makes a wonderful gargle for sore throats. Place 1 teaspoon of dried thyme in 1 cup of boiling water. Cover and steep 15 minutes. Strain and use as a gargle.

Chest Treatment

When spring comes, we often get spring colds. There are many herbs that can be of use to treat chest problems or to use as preventive care. Mullein, Irish moss, and horehound are all good herbs to keep on hand for the treatment of colds and chest congestion.

Asthma Tea

Simmer 1 teaspoon of ginger or cayenne pepper and 1 teaspoon of schizandra berries in 1 cup of water. Drink 2 to 3 cups daily. Do not drink if pregnant or breastfeeding.

Cold Sore Remedies

Cold sores seem to love sunshine, warmth, and moisture. The seasons of spring and summer have all the ingredients to bring on this painful condition. Here are a few treatments for that.

Sage Cold Sore Treatment

Add 1 teaspoon of dried sage to 1 cup of boiling water. Cover and steep for 15 minutes. Strain and add 1 teaspoon of ground ginger and 1 teaspoon of honey to sweeten. Drink 3 cups per day. You should have relief in about 24 hours. Do not use if pregnant or breastfeeding.

Thyme Cold Sore Treatment

Make a strong tea by adding 2 tablespoons dried thyme to 1 cup of boiling water. Apply as a compress to help relieve cold sores. Add several buds of balm of Gilead to help dispel pain and speed healing. Do not use if pregnant or breastfeeding.

Yogurt Cold Sore Remedy

Apply buttermilk or yogurt to the area to dry up the sore.

Stress Remedies

During mid-spring, we may be dealing with feelings of being overwhelmed or sensitive due to all the changes happening. Excessive emotional agitation can best be relieved by valerian, and the best way to use valerian is with a tincture. The body treats valerian exactly the same as valium but without the side effects. You should take precaution if you have heart or stomach issues. Instructions for making a valerian tincture can be found in chapter 8.

Hops Stress Relief

Hops can help you relax. Mix together 1 teaspoon each of hops, catnip, and chamomile. Store in a tightly closed container. Add 1 teaspoon of the mixture to 1 cup of boiling water. Cover and steep 10 minutes. Add honey to sweeten if desired. Drink as often as needed.

Mexican Marigold Tea

Mexican marigold has similar properties to marijuana. It is very relaxing when made into a tea. It has a pleasant taste and really needs no sweetener. Add 1 teaspoon of the dried leaves to 1 cup of boiling water. Cover and steep 10–15 minutes.

Skullcap Tea

Skullcap is great for nervous tension and is nonaddictive. Chop ½ cup of skullcap leaves and flowers and add it to 2 cups of boiling water. Cover and steep for 15 minutes. Strain and sweeten with honey. Drink several cups a day if desired.

Calming Herbal Tea

Mix together 1 cup each of skullcap, peppermint, and sage. Dosage is 1 teaspoon of the mix to 1 cup of boiling water. Pour the boiling water over the herb mix, cover, and steep 10–15 minutes. Strain and sweeten. Drink warm as needed to relax and to relieve headaches. Store the rest of the herb mixture in a tightly closed container. Don't use if pregnant or breastfeeding.

Sage Tea

Pour 1 cup boiling water over 1 teaspoon of dried sage. Cover and steep 15 minutes. Drinking this tea can bring an immediate sense of calm.

Passionflower Tea

Put several blossoms from a passionflower vine into 1 cup of boiling water. Cover and steep for 10 minutes. Strain and sweeten with honey.

THREE

Late Spring

MAY

We come to the tail end of spring, where the end is the summer solstice around June 21. Your ideas and energies are supercharged during this transitional time. We are usually healthy as we get settled into the season, but if you are the type that can wear themselves down to the bone, this time of the year is a concern. Excessive strain can cause lung problems to flare, which can cause blood disorders if you don't receive enough oxygen.

Herbs for Late Spring

Here are plants that I've categorized as healing herbs for late spring:

barley (*Hordeum vulgare*)

boneset (*Eupatorium perfoliatum*); do not use if you have liver issues.

calendula (*Calendula officinalis*)

camphor (*Cinnamomum camphora*); do not ingest.

comfrey (*Symphytum officinale*); do not ingest.

eyebright (*Euphrasia officinalis*)

fennel (*Foeniculum vulgare*)

horseradish (*Armoracia rusticana*)

lavender (*Lavandula angustifolia*)

mints (*Mentha* spp.)

parsley (*Petroselinum crispum*)

potatoes (*Solanum tuberosum*)

Queen Anne's lace (*Daucus carota*)

sage (*Salvia officinalis*); do not use if pregnant or breastfeeding.

scotch broom (*Cytisus scoparius*); only take in low doses.

skullcap (*Scutellaria lateriflora*); do not use if pregnant or
breastfeeding.

yarrow (*Achillea millefolium*)

Growing Your Own Foods

Balance is everything. If you have the interest, get into gardening
or some aspect of working with nature. It helps to balance us physi-
cally, mentally, and spiritually. The bonus is that you grow your own
herbs, fruits, and vegetables and know they are organic and fresh.

The fruits and vegetables good to eat during this time are asparagus, beans of all sorts, beets, brussels sprouts, carrots, cauliflower,
spinach, tomatoes, corn, celery, oranges, peaches, pineapples, plums,
bananas, apricots, and pears. Most of the vegetables mentioned are
blood cleansers or purifiers.

Tonics for Renewed Energy and Health

Tonics are good for giving the body a boost in health. They are like
concentrated vitamin shots, as the plants you use for them are pow-
erhouses of goodness.

Chickweed Tonic

Chickweed is an excellent blood cleanser and tonic for the whole system. It should be included in the diet of anyone with chronic conditions. By lightly steaming chickweed, it can be used as a spinach substitute. To make a tea, add 2 tablespoons of chopped chickweed to 1 cup of boiling water. Cover and steep for 10–15 minutes. Strain and drink once daily as long as desired. Chickweed should be taken only in low doses.

Watercress Tonic

Watercress is another great purifier. Add 2 teaspoons of chopped watercress to 1 cup of boiling water. Cover and steep 10–15 minutes. Strain and drink several times a day for about a week. Do not use if pregnant or breastfeeding.

Anemia Treatment

If you suffer from anemia, use this recipe to strengthen your blood. Mix 2 teaspoons of apple cider vinegar and 2 teaspoons blackstrap molasses with water or tea and drink daily to build up the blood.

Blood Builder

Another good way to strengthen the blood is with the following herb mix. You may need to dry the dandelion root to use year-round, and this is the time of year to harvest it. Add 1 teaspoon dried comfrey and 1 teaspoon dried dandelion root to 2 cups boiling water. Steep 10–15 minutes. Strain and drink after meals. Do not use if you have liver issues due to the use of comfrey.

Dandelion Tonic

This dandelion tonic is a great one to have on hand. Pick 1 ounce of dandelion flowers and wash well. Pour 1 pint of boiling water over the flowers. Cover and steep 10–15 minutes. Strain. Add an equal amount of honey and mix well. Take a daily dosage of 1 tablespoon to receive many of the vitamins and minerals your body needs.

Beet Tonic

Beets are a powerhouse vegetable packed with beneficial vitamins; try to eat some form of them once a week. Beets are an excellent blood builder. You can also make beet juice and gargle with it to treat sore throats. Canning beets is a good way to preserve and use the vegetable and its juices. If one learns to preserve their own food supply, they can have a purer and fresher product.

Lung Tonic

Yerba santa is a must to help heal and build the lungs during bronchitis, chest colds, or any other lung problem. Add 1 teaspoon to 1 cup boiling water and steep 15 minutes. Strain and sweeten. Drink warm several times daily.

Pleurisy Treatment

Vitamin A is great to treat pleurisy, so violet is a natural choice when making a tea for helping strengthen the lungs. Ginger can be added to soothe any stomach upsets or nausea. Start by mixing 1 tablespoon each of ginger, fenugreek, and violet leaves. Add 2 teaspoons of this mixture to 1 cup boiling water. Cover and steep 15 minutes. Strain and sweeten with honey. Drink warm several times daily. Violets also act as a sedative, so this tea is helpful when dealing with pain. Yarrow can be added for its pain-relieving properties, high potassium content, and antibiotic properties.

Cough Syrups and Drops

Many times, a cough syrup is needed to help expel mucus from the lungs during illness. Cough syrups can be made from one herb or a mixture of herbs. If prepared ahead of time, the syrup can be used year-round. I like to keep at least one ready for use. The time needed is minimal, and the cost is low. Because you are preparing your own mixture, you are sure of the purity of the product. Any of the helpful herbs can be added for different reasons. Do a little research into the properties of the herbs and make up your own recipes.

The base when preparing a cough syrup is a decoction. A decoction is a mixture that is boiled. There are a few basic rules to follow when preparing a decoction. Dried herbs are used, and after boiling the herbs to extract the needed properties (about 20 minutes), strain them out, add honey to the liquid, and simmer until the honey is well incorporated (about 2–3 minutes more). Flavoring can then be added. The mixture will thicken as it cools. Because honey is used, there is no need to add any preservatives. I refrigerate my cough syrups because taking the mixture when it is cold is more soothing to raw, irritated throats. The basic herbs to use include a stimulant or activator. An activator is an agent that temporarily increases functional activity. If a diaphoretic (something that causes perspiration) is wanted, add that along with an aromatic herb. These normally are antiseptic in nature, and they improve the taste. A demulcent (something that soothes and softens) is also generally added.

Cough Suppressant Syrup

Mix together 1 teaspoon each of dried boneset, wild cherry bark, slippery elm, yarrow, and elecampane root. Add 2 teaspoons Irish moss and ½ teaspoon thyme and mix. Then add 2 tablespoons each of balm of Gilead buds, mullein, and peppermint and mix well. Add the dried herb mixture to 1 quart of water and bring to a boil. Boil until the mixture is halved. Strain well and add 1 pint of honey. Simmer an additional 20–30 minutes. Cool and add flavoring. Wild cherry flavoring is really good with this blend of herbs. You can also add peppermint oil or any natural flavoring you enjoy. The mixture will thicken as it cools. Take as needed for coughs. Do not use if pregnant or breastfeeding.

Cough Syrup

Thyme is an excellent herb to use when treating coughs. Pour 1 pint boiling water over 1 ounce dried thyme. Try using lemon thyme for a better taste. Let steep 10–15 minutes and cool. Strain and add 1 cup of honey. It's helpful to warm up the honey in order to incorporate it well. Keep this mixture in the refrigerator. Dosage is 1 tablespoon several times daily for colds and coughing.

Cough Drops

It is very easy to make cough drops for sore throats and coughs using herbs. They don't contain chemicals, and you can use them on a daily basis. Any of the herbs that are helpful for sore throats can be used, but the most popular are horehound, lemon balm, peppermint, or slippery elm. Balm of Gilead bud is a great addition, as it has pain-relieving properties and a numbing effect to soothe the throat, but do not use if you are pregnant or breastfeeding. Nibble a small piece of the bud to see how it has a numbing effect in the mouth.

Simmer 1 cup dried herbs of any or several of the above herbs in 1 pint of water for 15 minutes. Strain and add 2 cups sugar. Boil until it spins a thread when you lift the spoon from the mixture. Drop the mixture by teaspoon into cold water to form cough drops. Drain and shake each cough drop in powdered sugar to keep them from sticking to each other. Wrap individually and store in a tightly closed container.

Another version is to mix 2 cups sugar, ⅔ cup of light corn syrup, and ¾ cup of the herbal tea desired. Boil for 2 minutes. Place a candy thermometer in the liquid and remove from heat when the temperature reaches 285 degrees. Do not stir until the temperature reaches below 260 degrees. Food coloring, citric acid for vitamin C, and flavors, such as wild cherry, can be added at this time. Less stirring causes less graining. Pour the mixture into molds and let harden on the counter. You can also make suckers with this recipe. It's great for children to have during illnesses because there is less of a choking hazard with a sucker than a cough drop.

Tea Remedies

You can't truly delve into herbalism unless you take a look at herbal teas and their medicinal uses. Find your favorite tea to keep on hand for minor ills you regularly encounter.

Cinnamon Tea

Cinnamon is a strong stimulant and brings out perspiration. It's good to drink when you have a cold. Simmer 6 sticks of cinnamon in 1 pint of water for about 30 minutes. Strain and sweeten with honey. Drink ½ cup warm as needed. Add milk to improve the taste.

Mullein Tea

Mullein is a demulcent and helps soothe sore throats. It is also a cough suppressant. Put a small handful of mullein flowers or leaves in 1 pint of boiling water. Cover and steep 15 minutes. Strain and sweeten with honey. Drink as often as desired.

Agrimony Tea

For persistent coughs, agrimony is a wonderful treatment. Agrimony is a plant from the rose family that bears slender flower spikes and spiny fruits. It is native to north temperate regions.

Pour 2½ cups boiling water over 1 tablespoon of dried agrimony flowers or leaves. Cover and steep until cool. Strain and use as a gargle to soothe sore throats. To use as a treatment for persistent coughs, take 2–3 tablespoons of the infusion in the morning and evening.

Kidney Diuretics

At this time of year, you may need a diuretic because you feel bloated or are holding water. There are many natural methods, but the two best for this are parsley and horseradish. Either is sufficient, and I have included both recipes. Try both when needed to find the one that works best for you.

Parsley Tea

You can use fresh or dried parsley to make this tea. If using dried, add 1 teaspoon parsley to 1 cup boiling water. Cover and steep 15 minutes. Strain and drink several times daily for treatment of kidney or bladder problems. If you are using fresh parsley, you will need to use a little more parsley as it is less concentrated. This is true of all fresh herbs. Place at least 1 tablespoon of fresh chopped parsley in the cup and pour 1 cup boiling water over the herb. Cover and steep 15 minutes. Strain and drink several times daily until symptoms are gone.

Horseradish Diuretic

Horseradish is another great diuretic, and it's a good mixture to have on hand if you suffer from frequent bladder or urinary tract infections. Pour 2 pints of boiling water over 1 ounce bruised mustard seeds and 2 ounces of freshly chopped horseradish root. Cover and steep 3–5 hours. Strain and place in a sterile bottle that closes tightly. Dosage is 3 tablespoons 3 times daily for about 2 days.

Sore Muscle Relief

All throughout spring we work our bodies after the winter's rest. We may have sore muscles or problems with our arms or hands. There are a variety of ways to use herbs to create remedies to relieve muscle aches.

Camphor Muscle Rub

Camphor blocks can be purchased at a drugstore or online. Shave the camphor square (1 ounce) into 1 pint of mineral oil in a pan. If mineral oil is not available, any oil that is not drying, such as vegetable, olive, or peanut oil, can easily be substituted. Place the pan in an oven on the lowest setting until the shaved camphor is dissolved. Pour into a labeled bottle for storage. Make sure to label that this is **NOT** to be taken internally. Camphor is very poisonous and should be kept out of reach of children. Use as an external rub as needed for sore muscles.

For sore arms and hands, adding menthol crystals to the camphor rub is the way to go. Menthol crystals can be purchased at a drugstore or online. The process is a little different from using only camphor; the oil does not need to be heated. Shave the camphor square (1 ounce) into a small glass bowl. Pour 1 ounce menthol crystals directly over the shaven camphor. Stir and set aside for 30 minutes, stirring occasionally. The menthol crystals react with the camphor, and they will dissolve into each other. When completely dissolved, pour the camphor-menthol mixture into 1 pint of mineral oil. Store in a labeled bottle, also marked for external use only, and rub on sore muscles. It is good for arthritic hands too. This liniment is great to treat chest congestion from colds or flu. Apply to the chest and cover with a flannel cloth to keep warm. It is very soothing and helpful.

Relaxing Baths

A bath to calm you after a busy day is easy to prepare and very relaxing. The basic preparation is to add ½–1 ounce of dried herbs to 1 pint of boiling water and steep for 30 minutes. Some of the herbs to relax you at bath time are chamomile, linden flowers, mullein, lemon balm, slippery elm, catnip, or lavender. Choose the herbs that are of a scent pleasing to you and experiment to find the ones most relaxing to you. Always strain the herbs before adding the water to the bath so you don't have a mess in your tub. Ginger or poplar bark can be added to a bath to promote circulation.

Lavender Bath Muscle Treatment

This recipe is for sore and overworked muscles, to relieve tension, and to help put one into a more romantic mood. The bath also relaxes you and is great for the skin.

Crush and mix 1 ounce of lavender flowers with 1 ounce of dried basil and 2 teaspoons of cinnamon. Place into a quart container and add 1 pint of witch hazel. Cover and place in a warm and sunny area for 2 weeks; shake daily. Strain and label the container. Add about ½ cup of the liquid to your bathwater for a relaxing time and to help ease sleep. This is also good to use to help bring down a fever.

You can make your own witch hazel. It is a shrub that is attractive, unusual in bloom, and easy to grow. The blooms come out in late winter and are bright yellow. It's a nice addition to your herb bed. Take ¼ cup of chopped witch hazel twigs or roots and cover with water 1–2 inches above the plant material. Bring the water and plant material to a simmer and gently cook for about 20–30 minutes. Watch carefully as the volume should reduce no more than half. Strain. There will be roughly ½ cup of witch hazel extract.

Apple Bath

Pour 1½ pints boiling water over ¼ cup of dried apple slices. Add ½ teaspoon each of cinnamon and whole cloves. Cover and steep 30 minutes. Strain and use as an addition to a lovely bath.

Lavender and Pine Soak

Mix equal parts of lavender and pine needles. Add to 1 pint of water and bring to a boil. Remove from heat. Cover and steep at least 15 minutes. Strain and add to a sudsy bath for a great soak.

Chamomile Wash

This is a good mix for washing infants as it is very gentle to the skin. It is also good for adults with dry and inflamed skin. Chop ½ ounce each of chamomile and fennel. Cover with plenty of cold water and steep for 30 minutes. Place this herb liquid on a low heat and bring the liquid and herbs to a gentle simmer. Cover and simmer for 10 minutes. Remove from heat and strain. Dip a washcloth into the liquid while warm and use to wipe a baby or child down. Adults can hand-wash their affected areas.

Bath for Aching Joints

Mix together 1 ounce each of burdock root, mugwort, sage, and comfrey leaf. Pour 1 quart of boiling water over the herbs and cover. Cover and steep for 30 minutes. Strain and add to bathwater as a treatment for arthritis and other joint complaints.

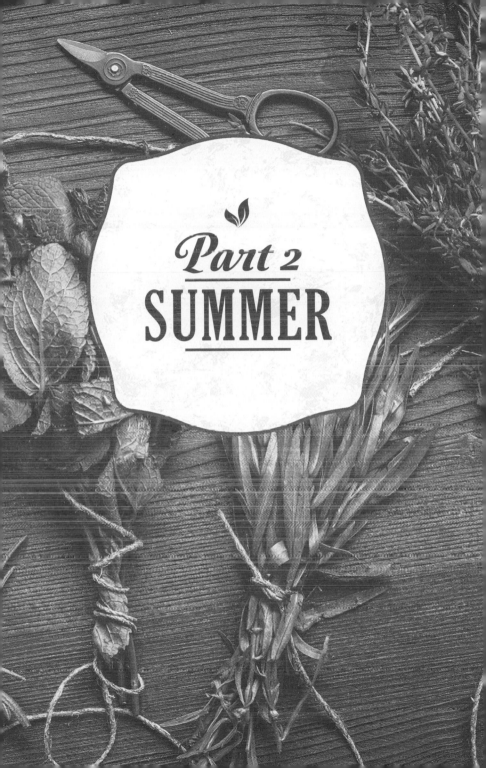

Part 2

SUMMER

FOUR
Early Summer
JUNE

Summer is a magical time. The summer solstice marks the longest day of the year. We revel in the sun as the birds sing. The plants are happily in full bloom, and the bees are busy buzzing around.

But there can surprisingly be a downturn in mood in the summer. Mentally, we may become dreamers who are brooding, scattered, and a little down. The sunshine and heat, though often associated with happiness and brightness, can be a trigger for anger and depression, and the summer can be a time when our moods and mental conditions suffer. According to Alison Jing Xu and Aparna A. Labroo, "On sunny days, depression-prone people also become more depressed. For instance, suicides peak in late spring and summer."[3]

Vitality may suffer as the hot sun beats down. Every little thing seems to loom bigger and feel worse. These negative feelings can upset the digestive system, and the stress can build to the point where there is a cascade of illnesses. The main problems at this time

....
3. Xu and Labroo, "Incandescent Affect."

of year are asthma and allergy problems, stomach and digestive issues, and nervous disorders. Healthy diets and working through gloomy thoughts will help keep your immune system running at peak condition so the body can heal itself.

Meditation is a good practice any time of year but especially in summer. It helps you be more grounded and makes delving into the problems of the spirit, soul, and unknown an easier exercise.

It is important to consume large amounts of green, leafy vegetables, as well as a variety of colorful vegetables, so you get all the vitamins and minerals your body needs. It is vitally important to your health that the diet be good and nourishing. Tonics work well for rejuvenating blood. Skin problems can result if the blood is deficient in certain minerals.

The best foods to consume for this time of year are eggs, rye flour, milk, cabbage, cauliflower, lettuce, watercress, pumpkin, blackstrap molasses, cheese, beans, spinach, clover, peas, carrots, squash, sweet potatoes, apples, peaches, and blueberries.

Herbs for Early Summer

Here are the plants that I've categorized as especially healing for early summer:

anise hyssop (*Agastache foeniculum*)
caraway (*Carum carvi*)
chickweed (*Stellaria media*)
dill (*Anethum graveolens*)
dock (*Rumex* spp.)
fennel (*Foeniculum vulgare*)
honeysuckle (*Diervilla lonicera*)
lemon balm (*Melissa officinalis*)

lettuce (*Lactuca sativa*)

marjoram (*Origanum majorana*)

nasturtium (*Tropaeolum majus*)

parsley (*Petroselinum crispum*)

peppermint *(Mentha piperita)*

potatoes (*Solanum tuberosum*)

red clover (*Trifolium pratense*)

sheep's sorrel (*Rumex acetosella*); use in low doses only.

spearmint (*Mentha spicata*)

St. John's wort (*Hypericum perforatum*)

Aromatherapy

Our moods can greatly affect our bodies and health. Essential oil is a concentrated oil extracted from a plant or herb that contains healing essences. Aromatherapy uses these essential oils and their healing essences to help with anxiety and mild depressive symptoms. There are three methods of aromatherapy that allow your body to absorb the healing quality of the oils: baths, inhalations, and lotions. These methods can begin to balance the body back into a healthier state. The following is a list of oils and what they can help alleviate. If the scent of one essential oil is not to your liking, you can exchange it for a scent you prefer.

Essential Oils for Anxiety

coriander: nervous weakness; sweet and uplifting

lavender: headaches and stress; soothing and relaxing

lemon: stress, nervousness, and feelings of being alone; use only in inhalations since it is a skin irritant.

melissa: tension; refreshing

orange: brightens mood, calms nervousness, and has an uplifting scent; use only in inhalations since it is a skin irritant.

rose: stress, headaches, and grief

sweet marjoram: tension; calming and warming

ylang ylang: anxiety; sedative

Essential Oils for Depression

basil: anti-depressive; uplifting and energizing

bergamot: mental clarity and uplifting

clary sage: nerve tonic for insomnia

geranium: balancing, uplifting

jasmine: relaxing and sedative

juniper: stimulating tonic

patchouli: sedative

Roman chamomile: insomnia

Aromatherapy Inhalations

For inhalations, the goal is to inhale the scent so the scented molecules from the essential oil enter your body through your nose. Place a few drops on a handkerchief to smell throughout the day or place a few drops on your pillow at night. You can use an essential oil diffuser to distribute the scent. For a powerful yet simple method, add a few drops to hot, steamy water in a bowl, cover your head with a towel, and lean over the bowl to inhale the steam. The goal is to use this therapy until you feel a change in your mood. It will help kickstart you out of the anxiety or depression you feel coming on.

Anxiety Inhalation

3 drops lemon

2 drops coriander

1 drop bergamot

Depression Inhalation

3 drops lavender

2 drops orange

1 drop geranium

Aromatherapy Baths

Aromatherapy baths are a great way to relax at the end of a stressful day, but they should be taken no more than twice a week. When creating the bath, you can just add the essential oils (6–10 drops) right to the bathwater, or you can use ½ cup Epsom salts to help disperse the essential oils.

Stress Relief Bath

3 drops lavender

3 drops melissa

Uplift Your Mood Bath

4 drops rose

3 drops Roman chamomile

Aromatherapy Lotions

Lotions not only keep our skin conditioned and looking smooth and glowing but they also help us absorb the healing qualities of the essential oils and help alleviate dark moods. Lotions are easy to make. Whip hardened coconut oil and castor oil in a stand mixer or with a hand mixer until smooth and creamy. Add your essential oils and mix well. Store in a glass container.

Uplift Your Mood Lotion
½ cup coconut oil

1 tablespoon cold-pressed castor oil

30 drops of your choice essential oil or a mixture according to your needs

Lavender and rose are my favorite for this purpose. Add fewer drops according to how strong you want the lotion.

Teas for Meditation and Stress Relief

Meditation has long been a way of refreshing your soul so you can face the world renewed. By learning to relax and not allow stress to rule our lives, we keep our system in a healthier state. Stress can lower your immune system so that you become vulnerable to many diseases. You then become more stressed because you are ill, and it becomes a vicious cycle.

Perhaps if we became aware of how closely our emotional state is tied to our physical health, we would be more willing to find ways to release stress. Often there is not much we can do to change the world we live in, and all we can do is learn new coping skills.

Thankfully in summer, fresh herbs are abundant and easy to find, and what faster way to relax than with a hot cup of tea—especially an herbal tea designed to sedate and calm us after a busy day?

Relaxing Tea

Mix together 1 tablespoon each of peppermint or spearmint, crushed fennel seeds, lemon balm, and hops. Place in a tightly closed container. Add 1 teaspoon of the mixture to 1 cup of boiling water.

Cover and steep 10 minutes. Strain and sweeten with honey. Drink about 30 minutes before bedtime.

Lettuce Tea

Lettuce has long been used as a sedative. The leaf-type lettuce is better than the head type, but use what you have in order to make the tea. Chop 1 cup of lettuce and pour 1 cup of boiling water over it. Cover and steep for 30 minutes. Strain and drink before bed for a relaxing rest. It can relieve tension and is good to use to unwind from a busy day.

Tension-Relieving Tea

Mix together 1 teaspoon each of dried peppermint, bruised caraway seeds, and dried lemon balm. Store in a tightly closed container. Add 1 teaspoon of the mixture to 1 cup of boiling water. Cover and steep 15 minutes. Strain and sweeten with honey. This tea is excellent to treat nervous tension.

Bay Leaf Tea

Many times, we can be our own worst enemy. When our imaginations get worked up and we get upset, this tea seems to work very well to calm down. Pour 1 cup of boiling water over 2 bay leaves. Cover and steep 10 minutes. Remove the bay leaves and sweeten with honey.

Rice Tea

Rice tea helps to soothe as well as settle upset stomachs. Place 1 cup of rice in 1 quart of water and simmer 10 minutes. Strain the rice from the liquid, saving the liquid. Add cinnamon and sugar to the strained water to flavor. Drink this beverage warm.

Peppermint Nervine

Mix 1 tablespoon each of dried peppermint, sage, and skullcap. Place 1 teaspoon of the mixture in 1 cup of boiling water. Cover and steep 10 minutes. Strain and add honey to sweeten. Drink warm every couple of hours as needed. This tea also soothes nervous headaches. If the tummy is upset, add ginger and fennel seeds to the mix.

Lavender Tea

Lavender is such a versatile herb, and a lavender tea will help dispel headaches, relax you, calm the mind, help with insomnia, and ease any tummy troubles.

To make the tea, add 4 teaspoons of fresh lavender flowers to 1 cup boiling water. Cover and steep 10 minutes. Strain. Sweeten with honey as needed.

Tonics for Stress Relief

Tonics are so important to your health, and I encourage you to take tonics even when you are feeling well. Many times, we overestimate our feeling of wellbeing and allow the immune system to get low enough to cause illness. If the immune system is healthy, our bodies are quite capable of fighting off disease and will help keep the system strong.

Nasturtium Tonic

This tonic benefits the blood and digestive system, and nasturtium is an easy plant to grow.

Put a small handful of nasturtium leaves and flowers into an earthenware bowl. Pour 1 pint of boiling water over the herb. Cover and steep for 30 minutes. Strain and drink several cups per day for 1 week. It makes a nice peppery drink and serves as a stimulant. The flowers and leaves also make a nice addition to salads for flavor and color.

Goldenseal Tonic

This recipe is particularly good for building energy. If your get-up-and-go has got up and gone, this replaces energy fast. Mix together 1 tablespoon each of goldenseal, cayenne pepper, and honeysuckle. Add 4 tablespoons of hawthorn berries. Store in a tightly closed container. Dosage is 1 teaspoon of the mixture to 1 cup of boiling water. Cover and steep for 10–15 minutes. Strain and sweeten with honey. Drink 1 cup daily for 1 week. Consult your doctor before using if you take heart medication.

Digestive Remedies

Because many of us often suffer from upset stomach, it's smart to have a few natural remedies for digestive aid. When we only use natural methods to treat simple upsets, we keep our system clear of chemicals that can add to an existing problem.

One of the most common rules when using herbs for digestive upset is to remember that any of the seed herbs can be used; anise, caraway, dill, and many other seeds are often used. Crush the seeds before preparing the teas. This allows your body to quickly get the properties needed from the seeds.

Dill Seed Tea

Bruise 2 teaspoons of dill seeds, including the chopped leaves if available. Cover with 2 cups of boiling water. Cover and steep until cool. Strain and sweeten. Drink about 2 ounces every hour until indigestion is alleviated.

Caraway Seed Tea

Mix together 1 tablespoon each of caraway seeds (has vitamins and minerals and helps with digestion), fennel (helps with acid reflux), aniseed (helps with digestive upsets), and coriander seeds (helps with gas). Substitute dill if you don't like one of the other seeds. Store the seed mixture in a tightly closed container. Bruise 1 teaspoon of the mixture and add to 1 cup of boiling water. Cover and steep until cool. Strain and sweeten if desired. Drink it warm or cold to help settle indigestion fast.

Parsley Tea

An herb can be used to treat more than one illness, and parsley is a good example. Not only does it treat indigestion but it also serves to flush the kidneys. You can use either dried or fresh parsley. Dried herbs are more concentrated than fresh, so you need to use less if using dried herbs.

Pour 2 cups boiling water over a handful of fresh parsley. Cover and steep until cool. Strain and sweeten.

Peppermint Tea

Peppermint has long been used as an aid for indigestion. Make a tea using 1 teaspoon of dried peppermint and 1 cup of boiling water. Cover and steep 10 minutes. Strain and sweeten with honey. Drink warm.

Marjoram Tea

Pour 1 cup of boiling water over several sprigs
of marjoram. Cover and steep 10 minutes.
Strain and sweeten with honey if desired.
This also serves as a treatment for headaches brought on by nervous tension.

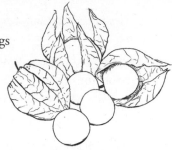

Digestive Aid

If indigestion is your problem, put ½ ounce powdered kelp into 2
cups boiling water and steep for 15 minutes. Drink as needed for
indigestion. This is an excellent way to absorb the iodine needed by
the body to stay healthy and strong.

Potato Tea

Perhaps you have allowed stress and tension to get the best of you
and you now suffer from ulcers. There are many treatments, but
one of the best is potatoes.

Boil potatoes and reserve the water. Let sit until it's cool enough
to drink. Drink at least 1 cup once daily for duration of treatment.

Red Clover Tea

This tea can be used for indigestion or for treating an ulcer. The
reason it is so helpful is because it helps to relieve excess acid.

Add 2 tablespoons dried or ¼ cup fresh red clover to 1 cup of
boiling water. Cover and steep 10–15 minutes. Strain and sweeten
with honey if desired. Drink 1 cup before meals and at bedtime.

Red clover has many minerals, so drink this tea anytime as a
tonic for the whole system. It acts as a blood builder and purifier.

Peppermint-Cranberry Tea

Hot weather calls for a nice cold drink. If you have nausea or indigestion, this tea will do the trick. The cranberry juice is an added boost for the kidneys to flush out toxins.

In a large saucepan, bring 4 cups of water and ⅔ cup loosely packed fresh peppermint leaves to a boil. Remove from heat and add 6 green tea bags. Cover and steep for 15 minutes. Discard tea bags. Cover and let stand 45 minutes longer. Strain and discard mint leaves. Stir 3½ cups reduced-calorie, reduced-sugar cranberry juice and 1 tablespoon lemon juice into the tea. Add sugar or honey to taste. Keep in the refrigerator for 4–6 days. Serve over ice with lemon slices if desired.

FIVE

Midsummer

JULY

July is smack-dab in the middle of the year, and it is a time of year we try to be most active, even though the weather can be a struggle. It is hot and steamy in some parts of the world, which is why many vacations are planned this month. Going to different places and meeting new people can up the risk for a summer cold and other ills. You may need help with nausea or vomiting if you find yourself fighting off some type of virus. An energy boosting may be much needed and appreciated at this time. It's common to need skin-saving remedies for sunburn, insect bites, and cuts this time of year as well.

Herbs for Midsummer

Here are the herbs I've categorized as especially healing for midsummer:

aloe vera (*Aloe barbadensis Miller*); only ingest in small doses.
apple (*Pyrus malus*)
black currant (*Ribes nigrum*)

boneset (*Eupatorium perfoliatum*)

borage (*Borago officinalis*)

calendula (*Calendula officinalis*)

comfrey (*Symphytum officinale*); do not ingest.

corn silk (*Zea mays*)

cranberry (*Vaccinium macrocarpon*)

ginger (*Zingiber officinale*)

ginseng (*Panax quinquefolius*)

goldenseal (*Hydrastis canadensis*)

hawthorn berries (*Crataegus oxyacantha*); do not use if taking heart medication.

holy basil (*Ocimum tenuiflorum*)

honeysuckle (*Diervilla lonicera*)

parsley (*Petroselinum crispum*)

peppermint (*Mentha piperita*)

rose (*Rosa* spp.)

rosemary (*Rosmarinus officinalis*)

sweet woodruff (*Galium odoratum*)

violet (*Viola odorata*)

Remedies for Chest Complaints, Allergies, and Asthma

If you suffer from chest complaints or asthma, your emotional state can be a contributing factor when it comes to breathing difficulties. When you are stressed, breathing becomes difficult and you take shallow breaths. It is a good idea to learn ways to relieve tension and restore balance to the system. An attack can be very frightening, so methods like meditation or breathing techniques can help you slow

down and calm yourself to lessen or help alleviate an attack.

If your asthma is caused by an allergic
reaction, there are many ways to help alleviate it. You can take allergy shots from
your physician or try a natural method.
Bee pollen is a great way to help ease
allergies. Bees in your region get pollen
from nearby plants that you may be allergic to,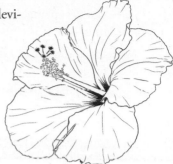
and the pollen can be used to slowly desensitize your system. Always
use care when treating yourself, especially when ingesting something
new. Consult a naturopathic doctor or other physician when using
this method, and start by taking a few grains daily, adding to the dose
until you can handle one capsule daily.

It's a good idea to start this treatment in December to slowly
desensitize yourself for when pollen season comes around in the
spring. Taking vitamin C during this treatment helps strengthen
your immune system. Taking B-6 twice daily during allergy season
will help too.

Honeysuckle Tea

Honeysuckle tea is a gentle relaxer for those who suffer from asthma.
Place 1 tablespoon of the grated root in 1 cup of boiling water. Boil
gently for about 10 minutes. Strain and sweeten with honey. Drink
daily to strengthen the system.

Fennel Seed Tea

Fennel seed tea has several uses besides being a treatment for indigestion. It is used by many as a treatment for asthma. Bruise 1
teaspoon each of fennel and fenugreek seeds. Pour 1 cup of boiling
water over the seeds. Cover and steep 15 minutes. The fenugreek

acts as a germicidal for the lungs and helps reduce inflammation. Do not sweeten if used as an asthma treatment; you can sweeten with sugar if used as a digestive aid.

Congestion and Cough Remedies

We all occasionally need a little help when it comes to summer colds and congestion. Try making these easy recipes with items you have on hand during the sunny days of summer.

Potato Steam Bath

The common potato comes to the rescue. Slice up several potatoes, place in a pot, and cover with water. Bring to a boil. Pour the water into a basin. Place a towel over your head and lean over the basin to inhale the steam for 5–10 minutes at a time.

Cherry Cough Treatment

Add a handful of cherry stems to 1 pint of boiling water. Cover and steep until the liquid is cool. Strain and add 1 pint of honey. Shake well and take 1 tablespoon as needed for coughing. Store in the refrigerator for up to 3 months.

Red Clover Cough Suppressant

Put 1 pint each of honey and water in a stainless steel pan. Bring the mixture to a boil and add 1 ounce each of red clover blossoms and lemon balm. Reduce to a gentle simmer for 10–15 minutes. Cool the mixture before straining. Place the water in a sterile bottle and keep refrigerated. Take 1–2 tablespoons of the mixture as needed for coughs.

Peppermint Congestion Treatment

Mix 1 cup of oil (vegetable, olive, almond, or peanut) and 2 teaspoons of peppermint oil and shake well. Massage the back and chest
area well with the oil. Cover your chest with a towel to keep warm.
Make yourself a cup of peppermint tea (the recipe can be found in
chapter 4) to drink. This produces perspiration, reduces fever, and
helps break up the congestion.

Anise Hyssop Tea

Hyssop leaves are used to grow the mold that produces penicillin, so
it makes sense to use the herb to treat colds, congestion, bronchitis,
and other related illnesses. Place several tablespoons of hyssop leaves
in a teapot. Cover with boiling water. Add grated orange or lemon
peel to the pot to make a very pleasant tea. Steep for 10–15 minutes
and strain. Sweeten as desired and drink hot.

Elderberry Tea

Mix together 1 tablespoon each of dried elderberry flowers, peppermint, and red clover. Place in a tightly closed container. Place
1 teaspoon of the mix in 1 cup of boiling water. Cover and steep
10–15 minutes. Strain. Sweeten with honey and drink warm, pref-
erably before bedtime. Use this rea to head off a cold you feel may
be coming on. The tea helps to stop it before it becomes a more
serious illness.

Cough Syrup

This cough syrup seems to help in cases of stubborn coughs. Mix
together 1 ounce each of hyssop, honey, horehound, and ground ivy.
Add to 1 pint of water. Simmer very low for about 1 hour. Steep until
cool and strain. Place in a sterile bottle. Take 1 tablespoon as needed
for coughs. Store in the refrigerator for up to 3 months.

Remedies to Fight Fatigue

Long summer days on the go and relentless heat can drain anyone's energy. Try these recipes to bring back a zip and zing to your step.

Ginger Tea

This spicy tea can banish fatigue and give you energy. Ginger is good for the adrenal glands, increases endurance, and helps the body cope with stress.

Combine 4 cups of water and a 2-inch piece of fresh ginger root, sliced thin, in a saucepan. Boil for 20–25 minutes. Strain, add the juice of ½ a lime or 6–8 drops of peppermint oil and honey or sugar to taste, and mix well. Store in a mason jar for up to a week. Makes about 4 servings. Serve over ice with a lime slice whenever you need an energy boost. You can double the recipe so you have more servings on hand.

Holy Basil Extract

Holy basil, also known as tulsi, is a sacred herb in Ayurveda medicine. It is an adaptogen, which is very balancing for the body and helps with stress. Both holy basil and rosemary are excellent for giving energy to the body. This extract will help the adrenal glands and is an anti-inflammatory boost for the immune system.

Fill a glass jar about halfway with holy basil leaves. Add a couple sprigs of rosemary. Cover with apple cider vinegar, making sure the vinegar covers the herbs by 2 inches or so. Place in a warm, dark place for up to 6 weeks. Shake daily. Strain into a small dark bottle with a dropper. Place 1 dropperful into your drink or under your tongue. You can do this daily for several weeks or whenever you feel you need a boost.

Summer Skin Remedies

Sometimes that hot sun can play havoc with our skin. When you have spent too much time outdoors and your skin is flaming, try these quick and easy home remedies.

Aloe Vera for Sunburn

The best burn or sunburn remedy is aloe vera. Having an aloe plant growing on your kitchen windowsill is so handy. With any burn, snap off a fat, juicy leaf and spread the gel on the burn to take away the sting. The gel is antibacterial and good for healing wounds.

Oatmeal and Baking Soda for Sunburn

After a long day in the sun, a soak in a cool tub with oatmeal and baking soda can heal and soothe. Put 1 cup of oatmeal and several tablespoons of baking soda into a thin fabric bag and toss it into the tub. Squeeze the bag to circulate all the healing qualities of the oatmeal and soda. Relax and soak in the water for 15–20 minutes.

Chamomile Tea Remedy

Chamomile soothes sunburn, helps heal wounds, and can reduce inflammation. Press a used, moist bag of chamomile tea onto affected skin. Keep it on the skin for 10–15 minutes as often as you feel the need. You can buy premade bags of chamomile tea or bag your own chamomile tea with ready-to-fill disposable tea bags.

Sunburn Salve

Calendula is one of the best herbs for treating skin issues like burns, inflammation, cuts, scrapes, bruises, bee stings, diaper rash, and eczema. It is antibacterial and anti-inflammatory. Lavender is also very healing for burns and is great for a wide variety of skin care. Use the two to make a salve that is easy to keep on hand for anytime you need something to help your skin.

First, you need to make an infused oil. Harvest and dry your calendula or lavender flowers. Fill an 8-ounce glass jar ¾ full with the dried flowers. Cover with an oil of your choice; use olive, almond, or jojoba. Place in a sunny window for 3–6 weeks and shake occasionally. Strain, and then make sure to squeeze the herbs to get all the oil out. Discard the used herbs.

Once you have made the infused oil, you will need to gather a double boiler and small glass jars or tins to make and store the salve. This recipe will make a little over 1 cup, or 4 2-ounce jars.

Add 1 cup of the infused oil and 4 tablespoons (1 ounce) of beeswax to the double boiler. Heat on the stove over medium heat until the beeswax is completely melted. Remove from heat. An optional step is to add 30 drops of essential oils of your choice to the mixture. For example, you can use 30 drops of lavender essential oil, or 25 drops of lavender essential oil and 5 drops of tea tree essential oil. Do whatever you like to the mixture as long as the total is only 30 drops per recipe. While still hot, pour the mixture into your containers, and let the mix solidify with the lids off until completely cooled. Apply the salve to skin freely as needed. Store it in a dark, cool place.

Natural Deodorant

Sunburn isn't the only thing to worry about at this time of year. Summer is a sweaty time. Using herbs as an odor preventive can be surprisingly effective. There are many ways even the most common vegetables or flowers can be used. Simply bruise a leaf of chrysanthemum or lettuce until you can squeeze a drop of fluid, which is chlorophyll, from the herb and into the palm of your hand. Rub this on your underarm to prevent odor. The chlorophyll destroys the bacteria that causes the odor.

During winter months, when fresh chrysanthemum leaf is not available, rub a drop or two of lavender essential oil on the area (use a carrier oil if your skin is sensitive) to prevent odor from developing.

You will still perspire using natural products, but the unpleasant odor will be gone. It is natural and desirable for the body to perspire.

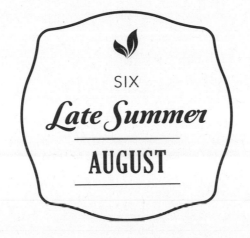

SIX

Late Summer

AUGUST

As the days of summer flow by, we come to the lazy, hazy time of year with plenty of time to dream and be creative. We may find ourselves overcompensating and trying to do too much or fit it all in before fall. If we do so, we have to watch over our hearts, spines, and generative organs. Climbing ladders, using lawn tools, and gardening can combine to overwork our bodies.

Herbs for Late Summer

Here are the herbs I've categorized as especially healing for late summer:

aloe vera (*Aloe vera*); only ingest in small doses.

angelica (*Angelica archangelica*)

apple (*Pyrus malus*)

caraway (*Carum carvi*)

chamomile (*Anthemis nobilis, Matricaria chamomilla*)

chickweed (*Stellaria media*)

costmary (*Chrysanthemum balsamita*)

cranberry (*Vaccinium macrocarpon*)

dandelion (*Taraxacum officinale*)

fennel (*Foeniculum vulgare*)

hops (*Humulus lupulus*)

horseweed (*Erigeron canadensis*); the young leaves are edible.

lettuce (*Lactuca sativa*)

licorice (*Glycyrrhiza glabra*); do not use if you have heart issues or high blood pressure.

nasturtium (*Tropaeolum majus*)

red clover (*Trifolium pratense*)

skullcap (*Scutellaria lateriflora*); do not use if pregnant or breastfeeding.

sweet woodruff (*Galium odoratum*)

violet (*Viola odorata*)

watercress (*Nasturtium officinale*); do not use if pregnant or breastfeeding.

Growing Your Own Foods

We all need to become self-sufficient in growing our own food supply so we can ensure that the foods we eat come from a healthy soil. I believe many of today's illnesses are directly related to the deficiencies in our soil. If you are unable to grow your own food supply, there are many local, organic gardeners happy to supply you with the fruits and vegetables needed for your health.

The Benefits of Gardening

An illness should not be treated as a single entity, and the focus should not entirely be on the body when treating an illness. The mind, body, and spirit should be treated with the same respect. Even if you treat physical complaints and are successful in relieving the symptoms, they will often return unless there is a change of mind and habits. Make sure your spiritual needs are met.

Learning to garden and supply your own food is a great way to relieve stress as well as treat the body for certain symptoms and get closer to nature. Don't worry if you don't have garden space. You can easily grow some herbs on your countertop or have a patio container garden. Either of these will get your hands in soil and get you closer to the plants.

We all need to take a look at our lives and realize that we aren't taking good care of ourselves when our lives get too hectic. The love we show to ourselves can help nurture and heal us of health-related tendencies our bodies may have.

A Quick Note about Magnesia

Magnesia is essential to our diet. Lack of it is shown through nausea, lack of appetite, diarrhea, loss of body coordination, tremors, and memory issues. It helps protect the heart, alleviates premenstrual syndrome symptoms, keeps blood pressure normal, helps prevent kidney stones and gallstones, can help prostate problems, and can alleviate indigestion.

The foods containing magnesia are barley, whole wheat, rye, almonds, lettuce, asparagus, cabbage, cucumber, walnuts, cranberries, garlic, onions, eggs, apples, figs, coconuts, and blueberries.

Heart Tonics

Because the protection of our heart is so important, let's turn to heart tonics. The tonics will not cure any heart disease, but they are helpful to your body and will allow it to better cope with any illness. The best way to protect your heart is to follow a healthy lifestyle and make sure you are receiving the vitamins and minerals needed for a healthy body. A lifestyle that includes rest and play, along with work and a stable emotional outlook, goes a long way in protecting the heart.

It is good to periodically take stock of your health, and the best way to start is with your heart. Here are some heart tonics to start your health journey.

Honeysuckle Tonic
Place 1 cup of grated honeysuckle root in 1 quart of water. Cover and simmer gently for 30 minutes. Strain and place in a sterile container. Refrigerate and drink 2 cups daily for 1 week.

Hawthorn Tonic
Fresh or dried hawthorn berries may be used to help your heart. Pour 2 cups of boiling water over 3 tablespoons of hawthorn berries. Cover and allow to sit overnight. The next morning, strain the berries from the liquid, and squeeze the berries to make sure you extract all the juice. Drink 1 cup in the morning and another in the evening. This treatment can be continued as long as desired. Do not use if taking heart medications.

Cardiac Tonic

Mix together 4 tablespoons of hawthorn berries (fresh or dried), 1 tablespoon of cayenne pepper, 1 tablespoon of goldenseal root, and 1 teaspoon of ginger. Store in a tightly closed container. Dosage is 1 teaspoon of the herb mixture added to 1 cup of boiling water. Cover and steep for 10 minutes. Strain and sweeten with honey. Drink several times a day for as long as desired. Do not use if taking heart medications.

Rose Tonic

Place a small handful of fresh wild rose petals or 3 tablespoons of dried wild rose petals in 2 cups of boiling water. Cover and steep for 15 minutes. Strain and sweeten with honey. Honey is a good tonic for the heart and should be used as a sweetener whenever possible. Rose hips can also be used for this remedy. Place 2 teaspoons of crushed rose hips in 1 cup of water. Bring to a boil and reduce heat to a simmer. Cover and simmer for 3 minutes. Strain and sweeten with honey. Drink several cups daily as long as desired. Rose hips are high in vitamin C.

Violet Tonic

Violets have long been used as a heart tonic. Macerate 2 teaspoons of violet leaves and add to 1 teaspoon each of ginger and goldenseal. Add the herb mixture to 2 cups boiling water. Cover and simmer gently for 15 minutes. Strain and sweeten with honey. This can be taken daily if desired.

Honey Heart Tonic

Mix 1 tablespoon each of ginseng, rosemary, hawthorn berries, and cinnamon into 1 pint of honey. Simmer gently for 30 minutes.

Strain and take 1 tablespoon every morning and evening. Do not use if you take heart medication.

Circulation Remedy

Perhaps circulation is your problem. One of the best ways to increase blood circulation is to prepare and take a capsule using common herbs. Every plant, vegetable, and fruit is considered an herb, and some people don't pay much attention to the more common vegetables and fruits as a treatment.

Apple Pectin Circulation Treatment

The ordinary apple is one of the better herbs that has long been underrated, and it's so important to incorporate apples into your daily diet. This recipe uses apple pectin, which you can buy or make yourself. Instructions for making apple pectin can be found in chapter 2.

Mix together 1 tablespoon each of apple pectin, lecithin, butcher's-broom, and cayenne pepper. Fill #00 capsules with the mixture and take 2 capsules in the morning and evening for about 1 week. Thereafter, take 2 capsules daily. You can take it as long as desired. This mix cleans the blood of toxins and helps when you have any circulation problems. It helps to take a vitamin B complex tablet when taking the capsules to amplify the effect.

Blood-Building Remedies

If you suffer from anemia, there are many herbs and treatments that you can use to strengthen the blood.

Bee Pollen Blood Building

Using bee pollen is one of the easiest ways to strengthen the blood. It is a biological stimulant that increases the red blood cells in the bone marrow and is available at your local health food store. The dosage is 2 teaspoons daily.

Dandelion Tea

Mix together 1 ounce each of dried dandelion leaf and fenugreek. Store in a tightly closed container. Add 1 teaspoon of the mixture to 2 cups of boiling water. Cover and steep for 10–15 minutes. Strain and add honey to sweeten. Drink after every meal.

Generative Organ Remedies

For minor ills related to the reproductive system, herbal remedies can come to the rescue. Summer is a time when problems of the generative organs often appear. High temperatures of the season can lead to dehydration and cause systems to not work optimally. As well, heat stress can bring on added disruption of hormonal balances.

Exercise caution when using these remedies; do not take them if you are pregnant.

Cramp Tonic

This is a good treatment for all menstrual complaints but especially cramps. Mix together ½ ounce each of orange peel, gentian root, and bruised coriander seeds. Mix the herbs with 4 ounces of brandy and allow to stand overnight. Add 4 ounces of water and allow to stand for another 12 hours, or overnight, before straining. Dosage is 1 tablespoon after meals.

Cramp Tincture

Prepare a tincture by placing 1 tablespoon of cramp bark and 1½ teaspoons each of ginger, yarrow, skullcap, cinnamon, and rosemary into ½ quart of brandy. Steep for about 2 weeks. Strain and place in a sterile bottle. Dosage is 1 tablespoon of the liquid added to 1 cup warm water. Drink as needed for cramps.

Blue Cohosh Treatment

Mix together ½ ounce each of blue cohosh, cramp bark, and skullcap. Place in 1 quart of brandy and steep for at least 3 days. Strain and take 1 tablespoon as needed for menstrual cramping.

Raspberry Tea

Nothing is better for menstrual problems than raspberry leaf tea. It adds the minerals needed to the system and aids in menstrual discomfort. It is also very helpful for the symptoms of menopause, as the tea acts as a sedative when your impatience gets the best of you during menopause.

Place 10 fresh raspberry leaves in 1 cup of boiling water. Reduce heat and simmer 10 minutes. Strain and sweeten. Use only freshly picked raspberry leaves; do not use leaves if wilted.

Menopause Treatment

Mix together 1 tablespoon each of motherwort, gentian, chamomile, valerian, ginseng, wild yam, and sage. Store in a tightly closed container. Add 1 teaspoon of the mixture to 1 cup boiling water. Cover and steep 15 minutes. Strain and add honey to sweeten if desired. Drink 1 cup daily to treat menopausal symptoms.

Menopause Tonic

Mix together 1 tablespoon each of skullcap, valerian, lavender, spearmint, and celery seeds. Store in a tightly closed container. Dosage is 1 teaspoon of the mixture in 1 cup of boiling water. Cover and steep for 10 minutes. Strain and drink warm. Drink several cups a day as needed and at bedtime.

Ginseng Treatments

This tea is great for energy and for those going through menopause. Many use it as a way to get some pep back in their step.

Know that daily use of ginseng can produce some side effects and can be dangerous for some people. If using as a tonic, only take it for 1 week at a time with several weeks of rest in between.

You can make a tea by adding 1 teaspoon of ginseng to 1 cup of boiling water and steeping for 15 minutes. Strain and add honey to sweeten.

The best way to take ginseng is in capsule form. This recipe gives you a lot of energy without the big dosage of ginseng by itself. Mix together 1 tablespoon each of ginseng, cayenne pepper, ginger, and violets. Fill #00 capsules and take 2 daily for 1 month. After 1 month, stop taking the capsules for 2 weeks, then take for another 2 weeks.

Pumpkin Seed Treatment

Use pumpkin seed to reduce inflammation of the prostate or bladder. This treatment is best if drunk as a tonic at least once a week. Put 4 ounces of pumpkin seeds in 1 quart of water and simmer 30 minutes. Remove from heat. Cover and steep until cool. Strain and drink several glasses a day.

Spearmint Treatment

This tea is good for relaxing the muscles of the stomach, relieving PMS symptoms, and for lessening discomfort from cramping. Place 1 tablespoon fresh or 1 teaspoon dried spearmint in 1 cup of boiling water. Cover and steep 15 minutes. Strain and sweeten if desired. Drink daily for 1 week.

Muscle Pain Relief

Many people suffer from muscle problems caused by overdoing it during activities like hiking, biking, swimming, or gardening during summer.

Muscle Liniment

Warm 8 ounces of cider vinegar. Mix together 1 tablespoon each of comfrey, cayenne pepper, and wormwood. Add the herbs to the warmed vinegar and steep in a warm area overnight. Strain. Melt a 1-ounce square of camphor and add to the liquid. Transfer to a jar for storage, shake well, and add a warning label to not drink. Rub the liniment on sore areas and place a damp, warm cloth over the area. Place a heating pad over the dampened cloth to keep the area warm. Rub the area every 30 minutes with the liquid and keep covered with the damp cloth and heating pad until relief is felt.

Boneset Poultice

Place ½ ounce each of dried boneset, comfrey, yarrow, and willow into 1 quart of water. Bring to a slow simmer for 15 minutes. Remove from heat and steep until cool. Strain and reheat. Dip a cloth into the liquid and apply directly to the area needing help. Keep warm with a heating pad. Replace this poultice every 15 minutes or so. Comfrey, willow, and yarrow contain the same properties as aspirin, so this poultice will affect the pain in a positive manner.

Sore Muscle Poultice

Mix together ½ tablespoon of cloves and 1 tablespoon each of mullein, chamomile, and boneset.
Place the mixture in a cloth and fold the cloth over
the herbal mixture. Place the folded cloth in very
warm water or apple cider vinegar. Wring out
sparingly so that it is not sopping with liquid
but still has good moisture. Apply directly over
the affected area. Cover with a flannel cloth and place
a heating pad over the cloth. Keep in place at least
1 hour.

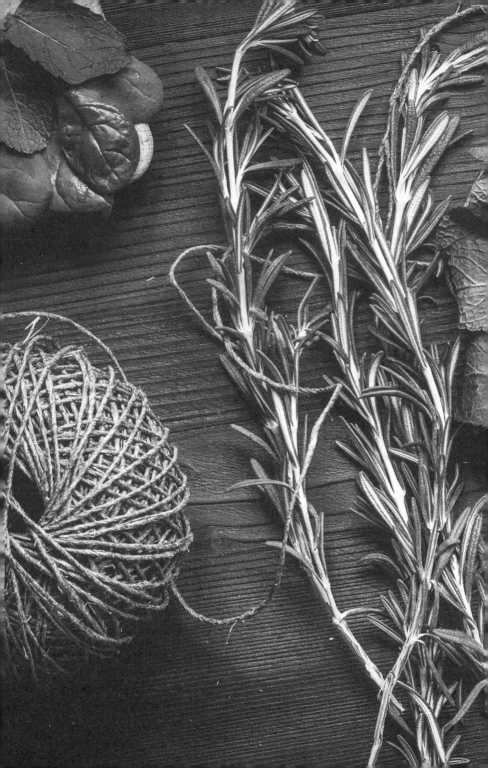

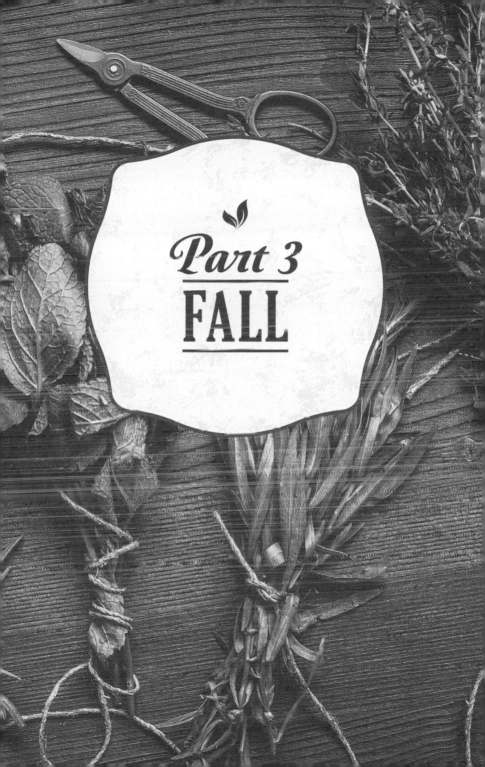

Part 3
FALL

SEVEN
Early Fall
SEPTEMBER

Fall is harvesting time. Pumpkins and apples are plentiful. Humans and animals alike are readying themselves for the coming winter. We celebrate all the bounty from our gardens, but often we can become materially minded this time of year. The tendency to prepare for the winter may become a hoarding for the winter, allowing our greedy sides to rear their ugly heads. With a balanced life and good health, we can often nip those tendencies in the bud.

Herbs for Early Fall

Here is a list of herbs especially healing for early fall:

apple (*Pyrus malus*)

burdock (*Arctium lappa*)

chamomile (*Anthemis nobilis, Matricaria chamomilla*)

chickweed (*Stellaria media*)

cranberry (*Vaccinium macrocarpon*)

fennel (*Foeniculum vulgare*)

feverfew (*Chrysanthemum parthenium*)

hops (*Humulus lupulus*)

nettle (*Urtica dioica*)

pansy (*Viola tricolor*)

parsley (*Petroselinum crispum*)

peppermint (*Mentha piperita*)

rose hips (*Rosa canina*)

sage (*Salvia officinalis*); do not use if pregnant or breastfeeding.

skullcap (*Scutellaria lateriflora*); do not use if pregnant or
breastfeeding.

thyme (*Thymus vulgaris*)

valerian (*Valeriana officinalis*); avoid if you have stomach or
heart issues.

violet (*Viola odorata*)

Skin Remedies

Skin problems are one of the warning signs that your diet is not balanced and you are lacking in vitamins and minerals. The skin regulates our body temperature and is our first defense against invading organisms. There are natural lotions and treatments you can make at home for personal care items that are free of chemicals.

Eczema Treatment

While eczema can be caused by internal as well as external conditions, look for external causes after you have corrected your diet and learned to deal with stress in your life. Stress and psychological factors can contribute to eczema. Meditation helps to control stress in daily living.

To make an external wash, place 2 tablespoons of pansies in 2 cups of boiling water. Cover and steep until cool. Strain and use as a rinse for the face daily.

Sun Damage Remedy

After a rough summer, your skin deserves some tender care for renewal. This recipe helps heal sun-damaged skin that is dried out and rough.

Mix together ⅓ cup each of rose water, glycerin, and lemon juice. Use after your bath or shower as a toner by rubbing it on you skin and leaving to dry.

Acne Treatment

Place 1 tablespoon each of dried willow bark or leaves and dried fennel in 1 cup of boiling water. Cover and steep until cool. Strain and use on the face daily.

You can add this liquid to a bit of plain yogurt and smear on the face for a mask. After you've applied the mask, place a hot washcloth over the face. As the washcloth cools, rinse it in hot water and replace it on the face. The moist towel helps the skin absorb the yogurt and its healing qualities. Wash off any remaining yogurt immediately afterward and pat your face dry.

Colored Bath Salts

Bath salts smell wonderful and are good for the skin. They are made with simple ingredients, including baking soda, Epsom salts, table or sea salt, essential oils, and coloring. Baking soda balances the natural pH of the skin, lowers inflammation, and is soothing for bug bites, acne, and blackheads, and the Epsom salts relax, remove toxins, and sooth sore muscles. The essential oils enhance the healing qualities; lavender is an all-around skin healer, tea tree is balancing and cleansing, and geranium helps clogged pores, eczema, and psoriasis. Adding color boosts the experience, and certain colors can bring good luck and enhance the mood.

The essential oils used can be homemade or can be purchased online or at health food stores. Rosemary and lavender are popular scents. Relaxing scents like lavender, geranium, bergamot, or rose will relax kids and help them sleep easier after bath time.

Some scent and color combinations work better than others. Peppermint or rosemary are good with green or pink coloring. The happy and bright citrus scents do well with yellow or orange coloring.

The ingredients needed to make bath salts can be mixed by hand or in a blender. Mix 1 cup each of baking soda, Epsom salts, and table or sea salt. Mix thoroughly and add a few drops of the desired food coloring and scent, then mix with the back of a spoon until the color is evenly distributed. Place in a plastic bag and seal. Exposure to air will harden the mix and dissipate the scent. Add 1 cup to the bath and enjoy!

Scalp Remedies

Fall is a good time to focus on your hair and scalp. We usually shampoo more in the summer than in the cooler months, and although there is no real seasonality to dandruff and scalp problems, they may become more apparent with the buildup of products and flakes as we head indoors. These issues can be dealt with in a natural way.

Dandruff Shampoo

This shampoo is easy to make and helps to control dandruff. It also acts as a stimulant, helping hair to grow. Place a handful of soapwort in a stainless steel pan. Pour 1½ cups of water over the herb. Bring to a boil and lower the heat to simmer. Cover and simmer for 10 minutes. Strain. Place in a tightly closed jar.

Put a handful each of red clover blossoms and chopped nettle leaves into an earthenware bowl. Pour 1 cup boiling water over the herbs and cover. Steep until cool. Strain and add to the jar of soapwort. Add about 4 tablespoons of castile soap flakes if desired. Shake well before each use. Keep refrigerated or in a cool, dark place for 10–14 days.

Scalp Rinse

To make a scalp rinse, place 2 tablespoons of the herb of your choice into an earthenware bowl. Pour 2 cups of boiling water over the herb and cover. Steep until cool. Strain and use as a final rinse after shampooing. Here are some herbs that make good rinses:

chamomile: lightens hair and promotes growth

fennel: a good conditioner

nettle: treats dandruff

parsley: helps clear up dandruff

rosemary: darkens hair and smells wonderful

sage: darkens hair and is a good conditioner

If you use a commercial shampoo, rinse with 2 tablespoons of apple cider vinegar added to 2 cups of water after you shampoo. Do not rinse out. This rinse counteracts any alkaline effects from the shampoo. Make the apple cider vinegar mix ahead of time, put in a squeeze bottle, and place it in the shower so it is always ready to use.

Immunity Tonics

When we take natural tonics, we are making sure our system is receiving the vitamins and minerals needed to fight foreign invaders like viruses and germs. Any of the natural substances not needed by the system are taken out through the urinary system and flushed from the body.

Red Clover Tonic

Add a small handful each of nasturtium flowers or leaves and red clover blossoms or leaves to a stainless steel pan. Pour 1 pint of boiling water into the pan. Cover and steep 30 minutes. Strain and drink several cups daily for about 1 week. The minerals and vitamins you receive from the clover make a wonderful tonic. Nasturtium is a great blood cleanser; it is also helpful for the digestive system.

Angelica Tonic

This tonic clears the urinary and bronchial system. Use it as an expectorant during colds. To make an angelica tonic, pour 1 cup of boiling water over 3 tablespoons of angelica. Cover and steep 10 minutes. Strain and drink warm. This tea is a stimulant and really picks you up when you are feeling tired.

Aloe Vera Tonic

The gel of aloe vera is used worldwide as a tonic for the whole system. It is a bowel regulator, and when the bowels are kept clear, the system can't absorb toxins. Add the gel of several aloe vera leaves to some water, about 1 cup, and mix in a blender until smooth.

Keep refrigerated, shake well before ingesting, and drink several sips daily if possible. Only ingest in small doses.

Cranberry Tonic

I believe nothing is better for your system than cranberry juice. It clears the bladder and kidney system, cleans the blood, and rids the body of excess toxins, all of which helps boost the immune system. Combine ¾ cup of 100-percent cranberry juice, ½ cup sparkling water, 1 teaspoon turmeric, and 1 teaspoon lemon juice. Stir until completely combined and add lots of ice.

Chickweed Tonic

This common plant is considered a pest to most people. It can be harvested from spring to early fall. You can lightly steam the plant and eat it as a side dish, add it to salads, or use it in other foods as a substitute for spinach.

Chickweed tea cleans impurities of the blood and acts as a tonic for the whole body. Place 1 tablespoon of fresh chopped chickweed in 1 cup of boiling water. Cover and steep 15 minutes. Strain and drink. Make this tea as often as desired. If you are using dried chickweed, remember to use less; dried herbs are in a concentrated form.

Chest Cold Treatments

The first few cold spells in fall, we may suffer from chest ailments. Chief among these problems are pleurisy and pneumonia. Neither of these illnesses are to be taken lightly. A physician's help is necessary. These remedies are to be used only until you reach help. It may be that it is the weekend, late at night, or some other time when you are unable to get in to see a medical doctor immediately. If it isn't an emergency, these treatments can help. If it is an emergency, get to the nearest emergency room or medical center immediately.

Pleurisy Treatments

Because pleurisy is an inflammation of the pleura, there will be sharp and intense pain under the rib cage. You can bind the rib cage to prevent pain when coughing or learn to hold your chest to prevent the pain. Lie on the side that is affected to prevent transfer of organisms to the unaffected area. Apply a warm or cool compress to the area to decrease the inflammation. Stay in bed and drink plenty of liquids.

You can also make a tea from thyme, yarrow, and fenugreek. Fenugreek is a germicidal for the lungs. It acts as a disinfectant and reduces inflammation. Thyme has antiseptic properties as well as expectorant properties. Yarrow has substances that are in aspirin. It's a pain reliever that also has properties, such as azulene, that fight inflammation and infections.

Mix together 1 tablespoon each of dried thyme, yarrow, and fenugreek. Store in a tightly closed container. Add 1 tablespoon of the mixture to 1 cup of boiling water. Cover and steep 15 minutes. Strain and sweeten with honey. Drink warm as needed.

Cough Remedy

Mix together 1 tablespoon each of dried thyme, balm of Gilead, Irish moss, mullein, and wild cherry bark. Place the mixture in 2 pints of water. Bring to a boil and reduce heat to a simmer. Simmer until the liquid is halved. Strain and add 1 cup of honey for every 1 cup of liquid. Simmer again for 15 minutes. Add peppermint or cherry flavoring. Take by tablespoonful as needed for coughs.

Red Clover Cough Syrup

Place 2 pints each of honey and water in a stainless steel pan and bring to a boil. Reduce heat to simmer and add 2 ounces of red clover blossoms, 2 tablespoons of balm of Gilead, and 2 tablespoons of mullein. Simmer for 15 minutes. Cool, strain, and place in a sterile bottle. Refrigerate and give 1–2 tablespoons for coughs as needed.

Pneumonia Compress

There are over 50 different causes for pneumonia, and this is one illness you don't want to fool around with. Get help as soon as possible. Until help is reached, I would suggest this garlic treatment.

Mash 1 head of garlic. Place in 2 cups of water. Bring the water to a boil. The fumes should be very strong. If at all possible, have the patient in the room while preparing the mixture. Dip a clean cloth in the liquid and apply it to the chest area. Be careful to not burn the skin. As the cloth cools, remove and repeat the procedure. Place some of the crushed garlic in a jar and pour boiling oil over it. Keep the jar tightly closed and allow the patient to smell the mixture every so often. If they can eat, have them chew small pieces of garlic during the treatment, or make them a garlicky broth to drink.

Diaphoretic

This tea helps to bring down high fevers and aids in eliminating toxins from the system. Diaphoretics should be used in moderation as too much can exhaust the patient. Take only until the desired result is obtained.

Mix together 1 teaspoon each of elderflowers, boneset, yarrow, and peppermint. Store in a tightly closed container. Place 1 teaspoon of the mixture in a cup and pour 1 cup of boiling water over the herbs. Cover and steep 10 minutes. Strain and sweeten with honey. Drink warm every hour or until perspiration is activated and the fever begins to come down. The elderflowers stimulate the secretion of the sweat glands.

EIGHT

Mid-Fall

OCTOBER

Now we come to the middle of the fall season. The harvests are mostly done, and the larders are filled. This is a time to stand back in the luxury of knowing you have prepared for winter. It's time to pull out the cozy quilts and sweaters and light fires to warm the bones on those dark nights.

Because we are indoors more, germs and illnesses can easily spread. Foods that are important this season are celery, carrots, spinach, beets, asparagus, peas, corn, wheat, rice, almonds, strawberries, apples, figs, raisins, blueberries, and coconuts.

Herbs for Mid-Fall

Here is a list of herbs especially healing for mid-fall:

apple (*Pyrus malus*)
burdock (*Arctium lappa*)
coltsfoot (*Tussilago farfara*); avoid if you have liver issues.
comfrey (*Symphytum officinale*); do not ingest.
ginseng (*Panax quinquefolius*)

horehound *(Marrubium vulgare)*

hyssop *(Hyssopus officinalis)*

Irish moss *(Chondrus crispus, Gigartina mamillosa)*

licorice *(Glycyrrhiza glabra)*; do not use if you have heart issues or high blood pressure.

marsh mallow *(Althaea officinalis)*

mullein *(Verbascum thapsus)*

peppermint *(Mentha piperita)*

rose *(Rosa canina)*

sassafras *(Sassafras albidum)*

wild strawberry *(Fragaria virginiana)* and garden strawberry *(Fragaria vesca)*

willow *(Salix* spp.)

Healing Tonics

There's a lot to love about mid-autumn: the crisp leaves, the brisk air. The cold winds start to blow, and we often begin to long for everything cozy: excess food, comfy chairs, and less exercise. But let's not become too self-indulgent; we have to keep our bodies in tune. Let's look at some tonics that are good for keeping the body balanced.

Strawberry Tonic

Wild strawberry leaf tea holds many minerals we so desperately need. It is easy to dry these leaves for use all year around. Drinking the tea several times daily for 1 week out of each month is a good practice. To make the tea, pour 1 cup of boiling water over 1 teaspoon of the dried leaf, cover, and steep 15 minutes. Strain and sweeten with honey. Drink 2–3 times daily for 1 week.

Rose Hip Tonic

Rose hips make a wonderful tonic, and the tea is good to drink when suffering from a cold or the flu. Chop 2 teaspoons of dried rose hips and add 2 teaspoons of dried violet leaves or flowers. Pour 1 cup of boiling water over 2 teaspoons of this mixture. Cover and steep 15 minutes. Strain and sweeten with honey. Drink daily for as long as desired.

Parsley Tonic

If treating a kidney or bladder infection, there are many herbs you can use, but parsley is one of the best. Anytime you need to take a diuretic, it is important to replace the loss of potassium. You can do this by adding yarrow to any natural treatment you are using. Yarrow has pain-relieving properties, and it's a good source of potassium.

Using dried herbs, mix together 1 tablespoon each of parsley, yarrow, and peppermint. Store in a tightly closed container. Add 2 teaspoons of the blend to 1 cup of boiling water. Cover and steep for 10–15 minutes. Strain and drink up to 4 times daily for a week for urinary tract infections.

Tinctures

Tinctures are great for mid-fall because they have a long shelf life compared with remedies preserved through other methods. That means your tincture remedy will last throughout the season, through winter, and possibly beyond. Preparing a tincture only requires a small amount of the herb(s), too, and the small bottle of tincture doesn't take up much room. Detailed instructions for making tinctures can be found in appendix A.

Valerian Tincture

Valerian is one of the better relaxants. I use it most frequently by preparing a tincture. Use either powdered or chopped valerian root and place the herb in a jar. Cover the herb with vodka and place in a warm, sunny area for about 2 weeks. Strain and place in a sterile jar. Most people don't like the odor of valerian, and this tincture does not improve the smell. I take it by placing several drops under the tongue. This tincture is good for anything from headaches to nervous tension, and it does help you to get a good night's rest. The tincture can also be used externally on poison ivy and other skin disorders.

Tinctures are easy to carry with you, making them especially helpful if you use them to treat colds or other simple illnesses. I make a peppermint tincture to carry with me in case someone has an upset stomach or heartburn. Taking this valerian tincture with you to work can help with a particularly stressful day. Simply add a few drops to your coffee or tea to calm jittery nerves.

Skullcap Tincture

To get rid of a nagging headache or to treat the flu, mix equal amounts of skullcap, thyme, and hops. Place in a jar and cover completely with alcohol or water. Place in a pot of water, bring the water to a boil, and boil for 15 minutes. Strain and add a preservative if needed. Place in a sterile jar and label. Dosage is 3–4 dropperfuls in 1 cup of boiling water to make a tea. You can add the tincture to juice or a small amount of water if desired. Skullcap and hops are both great relaxers. Thyme is a great astringent and will help with the flu.

Willow Tincture

Make a tincture, as directed in Skullcap Tincture recipe, using the twigs, leaves, or bark of a willow tree. Take to relieve pain.

Muscle Relief

As the days begin to shorten, we often have a tendency to overdo as we try to enjoy the last few warm days of the season. This can lead to aches and pains. Whether we overexercised and got sore, strained a muscle, or simply have an aching back, it is very convenient to have a home remedy on hand to ease the trouble.

Peppermint Liniment

A great liniment for tight muscles can be made with peppermint. Add 1 cup of peppermint leaves to ½ pint of oil of your choice. Place in a double boiler on low heat and let the oil warm slowly. The warmed oil should steep 15–30 minutes—until you can smell peppermint strongly. Strain out the leaves, add 2 teaspoons of lanolin, and stir until melted. Remove from heat. Stir continuously until creamy in consistency. Store in a tightly sealed container in a cool, dark place. Use as a rub for backaches, sore muscles, or arthritis.

Poultices

A poultice is nothing more than an external way to treat sore and aching muscles, swelling, sprains, gout, or congested lungs. Prepare a very strong tea using any of the appropriate herbs, or wilt the herbs down and place directly on the area needed. If the area is small, dip a cloth or piece of bread in the strong tea and apply to the area. This keeps the liquid in contact with the skin; the bread molds itself to the body part being treated.

Buttermilk Treatment

A good treatment for pulled muscles in the back is to dip a flannel cloth in warmed buttermilk and apply the cloth to the back. Cover the cloth with plastic wrap to hold in the heat and apply a heating pad. Replace with a freshly dipped cloth every so often.

Horseradish Poultice

This simple poultice really works well for back pain and arthritis. Grate a fresh horseradish root and moisten slightly with water. Place the damp root in a porous cloth and fold over. Apply to the area needed for pain relief.

Kidney and Bladder Relief

Sometimes we experience kidney or bladder problems and can't get to the doctor in a timely manner. To prevent these problems or to ease the symptoms until you reach a doctor, try these remedies as we continue through the autumn season.

Diuretic Tea

This tea helps when you are suffering with back pain caused by kidney problems. Mix together 1 tablespoon each of corn silk, skullcap, hops, yarrow, and willow bark. Store in a tightly closed container. Add 1 teaspoon of the herb mixture to 1 cup of boiling water. Cover and steep 15 minutes. Strain and sweeten with honey. Willow and yarrow are both pain relievers. Yarrow replaces any loss of potassium caused by the use of corn silk, which is a strong diuretic. Skullcap and hops are great relaxers. Drink as needed for pain and kidney infections.

Rose Hip Treatment

Rose hips help when you are having bladder problems. Crush 1 tablespoon of rose hips and add to 1 cup of boiling water. Cover and steep 15 minutes. Strain and sweeten with honey. Drink as often as desired.

Urinary Tract Treatment

To treat the whole system, place 1 tablespoon each of pansy, thyme, and parsley in 2 cups of boiling water. Cover and steep 15 minutes. Strain and sweeten with honey if desired. Use daily for 1 week.

Kidney Stone Treatment

At some time in your life, you may be troubled with kidney stones. To help pass the stones, mix together 1 teaspoon of dried parsley and 4 tablespoons each of lemon juice and olive oil. Add 1 tablespoon of the mixture to 1 cup of boiling water. Drink daily for 1 week.

Cucumber and Carrot Juice Treatment

The combination of cucumber juice and carrot juice is a great treatment for the kidneys. It removes the excess uric acid from the body and adds potassium to your system at the same time. Simply juice both a cucumber and a carrot and drink a glass daily to improve your health.

Fennel Tea

Fennel tea is great to drink as it flushes the kidneys and can prevent backaches from kidney problems. Add 1 teaspoon of crushed fennel seeds to 2 cups of boiling water. Cover and steep until cool and strain. Drink 2 cups daily for 2–3 days.

Burdock Root Tea

Burdock root is a great tonic for the whole system and an excellent diuretic. Add 1 teaspoon each of crushed burdock seeds and thyme leaf to 1 cup of boiling water. Cover and steep 15 minutes. Strain and sweeten with honey. Thyme is an excellent astringent, so it works to clean the kidney and bladder. Drink 1 cup daily for 1 week as a treatment.

Boneset Plaster

Boneset has long been used as an aid in healing broken bones, and a plaster is an excellent way to prevent or treat back pain. Place a very large handful of fresh boneset in 1 quart of boiling water. Cover and steep until the herb is wilted. Remove the herb from the water and place in a clean cloth that has been dipped in the liquid; the cloth shouldn't be dripping but plenty moist. Rub cold-pressed castor oil on the back area and place the boneset plaster on the painful area. Place a plastic wrap over the plaster and apply a heating pad to keep the plaster warm. Leave in place for 30 minutes. Repeat once daily until relief is obtained. This treatment will often make you need to go to the bathroom soon after the plaster is removed. This is good because a backache can also be caused by failure to keep the bowels moving freely.

NINE

Late Fall

NOVEMBER

As the season slides into late fall, the tendency toward excess can continue. Not only in feelings of needing more but in overwork. Instead of overworking, perhaps we can finally give ourselves permission to take care of ourselves so we can protect our health now and in the future—everything adds up. As Mary Ellen Carter and William A. McGarey write in *Edgar Cayce on Healing*, "Physical and psychological trauma, the aging process, the residuals of previous illness, improper dietary habits, the stress and strain of life decisions, all these contribute to illness in a multitude of ways."[4]

Problems that pop up in late fall often have to do with the generative organs. Bladder problems may also be a concern.

Foods particularly important this time of year include onions, garlic, mustard greens, cress, turnips, kale, asparagus, cauliflower, leeks, radishes, figs, prunes, black cherries, gooseberries, blueberries, and coconuts.

. . . .
4. Carter and McGarey, *Edgar Cayce on Healing*, 170.

Herbs for Late Fall

Here is a list of herbs especially healing for late fall:

apple (*Pyrus malus*)

chamomile (*Anthemis nobilis, Matricaria chamomilla*)

chicory (*Cichorium intybus*)

comfrey (*Symphytum officinale*); do not ingest.

dandelion (*Taraxacum officinale*)

hawthorn berries (*Crataegus oxyacantha*); do not use if you are taking heart medication.

hyssop (*Hyssopus officinalis*)

nettle (*Urtica dioica*)

oak (*Quercus* spp.)

parsley (*Petroselinum crispum*)

primrose (*Primula vulgaris*)

red clover (*Trifolium pratense*)

sassafras (*Sassafras albidum*)

Soloman's seal (*Polygonatum officinale*)

wild strawberry (*Fragaria virginiana*) and garden strawberry (*Fragaria vesca*)

valerian (*Valeriana officinalis*); avoid if you have stomach or heart issues.

violet (*Viola odorata*)

willow (*Salix* spp.)

A Quick Note about Potassium

Summer is now far behind us, and autumn begins to draw to a close. The days are getting shorter and shorter, and the sun is beginning to wane. It is important to make sure we head into winter with a balance of vitamins and minerals in order to keep the body strong. One very important mineral for the body is potassium. Lack of this vital mineral affects the liver and bile secretions and affects the scalp with hair loss or thinning hair. Dandruff may be noticeable.

Including plenty of fresh fruits and vegetables in your diet is the best way to receive the most potassium. Foods containing important vitamins and minerals that you should include in your diet are endive, chicory, carrots, whole wheat, oats, rye, avocado, cabbage, celery, all salad vegetables, pears, bananas, grapes, cantaloupes, and oranges.

Licorice (*Glycyrrhiza glabra*), which is a member of the legume family, should be included as well as various types of beans and peas. Licorice has shown to be effective in inhibiting disorders of the immune system. However, there are cautions that need to be added with the use of licorice. Too much consumption of the root can cause a disturbance in the balance of potassium and magnesium chemistry in the body, resulting in serious adverse effects for the heart. With moderation, licorice is useful in the prevention and treatment of high blood pressure. It protects against strokes and stroke-related deaths.

Menopause and Menstruation Remedies

Let's talk about menopausal symptoms. If you begin a natural treatment when symptoms first appear, you can often avert some of the more severe symptoms. Wild yam is one of the more important herbs we can use for this. It nourishes both the adrenal glands and the ovaries. Once the ovaries quit producing estrogen, the adrenal glands are supposed to pick up the slack and begin producing estrogen. By using wild yam, licorice root, and black cohosh root, the ovaries stay healthy much longer and the adrenal glands are taught to pick up where the ovaries left off.

Menopausal Treatment

Menopause symptoms include nervousness, irritability, restlessness, headaches, and sleep disorders. To help with those symptoms, several sedative herbs are included in this treatment. Using the powdered forms, mix together 1 tablespoon each of black cohosh, wild yam, licorice root, skullcap, valerian, and chamomile. Motherwort can also be added as it strengthens the nerve system and relieves menstrual discomforts. Mix thoroughly and place in #00 capsules. Take 3 capsules daily until symptoms abate. You can then reduce the dosage to 2 capsules daily.

Energy Treatment

Overworking often depletes us of energy, especially if we are experiencing perimenopause or menopause. There are many herbs we can take to increase stamina and receive extra energy. Mix together

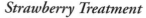

1 tablespoon each of ginseng, cayenne pepper, and gotu kola. Fill #00 capsules and take 2 capsules 3 times a day for about 1 month. Stop for 2 weeks and begin taking the capsules again for another month.

Strawberry Treatment

Strawberry leaves and willow make a good tea to drink for painful menstruation. Mix together 1 tablespoon each of willow bark and dried strawberry leaves. Store in a tightly closed container. Add

1 teaspoon of the mixture to 1 cup of boiling water. Cover and steep 15 minutes, then strain. Sweeten if desired. Drink as needed.

Apple Treatment

Apples are packed with antioxidant nutrients that can help ease symptoms of menopause. To clean the whole system, drink apple tea as often as you desire. The taste is pleasant, and the tea is easy to make. Place several slices of dried apple in 1 cup of boiling water. Add ½ teaspoon of cinnamon. Cover and steep 15 minutes. Drink as often as desired.

Raspberry Treatment

Raspberry leaf tea is an excellent way to get many needed minerals in your system during menopause. By adding red clover blossoms, you double your mineral intake. Place 1 teaspoon each of red clover blooms and dried raspberry leaves in 1 cup of boiling water. Cover and steep 15 minutes. Strain and add honey to sweeten.

Prostate Relief

The prostate can often experience a flare-up in the fall. Here are some recipes to maintain a healthy prostate.

Pumpkin Treatment

Pumpkin seeds are well known for their ability to restore healthy function of the prostate gland. Those with a prostate should develop a habit of drinking pumpkin tea at least once weekly and munching on pumpkin seeds to prevent prostate problems later in life.

Add 4 ounces of pumpkin seeds to 1 quart of water. Cover and simmer for 30 minutes. Remove from heat and steep until cool. Strain. Drink 1–2 glasses once a week.

Cucumber Treatment

Another good prostate treatment is to drink plenty of cucumber juice. Cucumber juice can also reduce high blood pressure when mixed with carrot juice. Include plenty of these vegetables in your daily diet if unable to extract their juice. If you suffer from gout, this mix of juices will also help remove the excess uric acid from the system.

Burdock Tonic

Burdock root has anti-inflammatory properties and is good for prostatitis, which is inflammation of the prostate. Place ¼ cup of dried burdock root in 1 quart of water. Bring to a gentle boil. Cover and simmer for 30 minutes. Remove from heat and add 1 tablespoon of meadowsweet flowers. Cover, steep until cool, and strain. Drink 1 glass daily for 3–4 days as a tonic.

Rose Tonic

Used in a tonic, roses can't be beat. Rose tonics contain a natural form of vitamin C, which acts as an immune booster. Add 3 teaspoons of crushed rose hips to 1 cup of water. Bring to a slow boil. Cover and boil gently for 3 minutes. Remove from heat and strain. Sweeten with honey. Drink 4 times daily for 2 days as a tonic.

Cleansing Tonics

Tonics, especially cleansing tonics, are incredibly helpful in the spring and fall. It is through the urinary tract and skin that toxins leave the system. We need to keep our systems flushed in order to expel all toxins, and it is important to keep bacteria from forming in the urinary tract. By drinking plenty of fluids daily, we can help prevent bladder problems. Here are recipes for tonics to help clear the system and rid it of toxins.

Corn Silk Treatment

Corn silk is an excellent way to treat bladder and kidney infections. Use this treatment once a month to clean the urinary tract. The addition of yarrow is to replace the potassium lost when taking this treatment. Add 1 tablespoon of dried corn silk and 1 teaspoon of dried yarrow to 2 cups of boiling water. Cover and steep for 15 minutes. Strain and drink several times daily for 2 days.

Ginseng Treatment

Ginseng has long been used as an herbal remedy because it helps maintain normal blood sugars and supports cognitive functions and energy and stamina. It tones up the system, so it helps in all areas. Many take it in capsule form. If taking ginseng as a tonic, fill #00 capsules with ginseng powder and take 2 daily for 1 month. Skip for 1 month, and then take for another month.

Blackberry Bath Tonic

Blackberries are good to eat and excellent for you internally, and the leaves can be added to the bathwater as a soaking tonic. Place a handful of blackberry leaves in 2 cups of boiling water. Cover and steep 15–30 minutes. Strain and add to the bathwater for an invigorating soak.

Borage Tonic

Borage is a great tonic that stimulates the adrenal glands. They release adrenaline in the bloodstream to give you extra energy. Chop 2 tablespoons of borage leaves or flowers and add to 2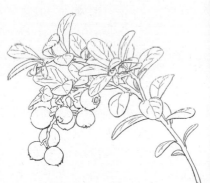

cups of boiling water. Cover and steep 10–15 minutes. Strain and drink several cups daily for 1 week.

Super Tonic

The stronger your immune system, the easier it is to hold off colds and chest complaints. If you keep a balanced diet, you are less apt to suffer frequent illnesses. The whole reason for using natural products is to build up the immune system and keep chemicals and synthetics out of your system. Our bodies fight daily against toxins in the atmosphere and air we breathe. We can be subjected to toxins at our workplaces and at home. This recipe makes a great tonic that removes toxins from the system. The ingredients are often easy to find or purchase, and it is easy to prepare.

Mix together 6½ cups of burdock root, 1 pound of sheep's sorrel, 1 ounce turkey rhubarb root, and ½ cup, by scale weight, of slippery elm. Store in a tightly closed container. Place 1 cup of the mixture in 1 gallon of boiling water. Cover and boil 10 minutes, then remove from heat. Scrape the sides of the pan down and stir well. Replace the cover and boil for an additional 20 minutes. Strain several times before pouring into sterile bottles. Store in the refrigerator. The dosage is 4 tablespoons of the liquid to 4 tablespoons of warm water. Take on an empty stomach daily before bedtime as a tonic to build the immune system.

Sheep's Sorrel Water

Used for a wide variety of ills, sheep's sorrel water is cleansing, boosts the immune system, and helps various organs of the body to function properly. Take a quart bowl and fill it ⅔ full of green sheep's sorrel. Cover with water and let stand for 1 hour. Mash to get the strength of the herb. Strain and pour into a mason jar with a lid to store in the refrigerator. Drink a small amount once daily. Only ingest it in small doses. You can use dried sheep's sorrel, but with that you must use boiling water and allow it to steep in order to extract the ingredients from the herb.

To use on an open sore, make a poultice by soaking the fresh sheep's sorrel in warm water until wilted and soft. Place on the sore. Change the poultice often.

Respiratory Tonic

Mix 1 ounce each of marshmallow root, licorice root, hyssop, and slippery elm. Pour 2 pints of water over the herbs. Cover and simmer until the liquid is reduced to half. Strain and drink ½ cup of the liquid every couple of hours 1 day a week for 1 month. This tonic nourishes and stimulates the adrenal glands, and it is a great tonic to build up the lungs and the respiratory system as a whole.

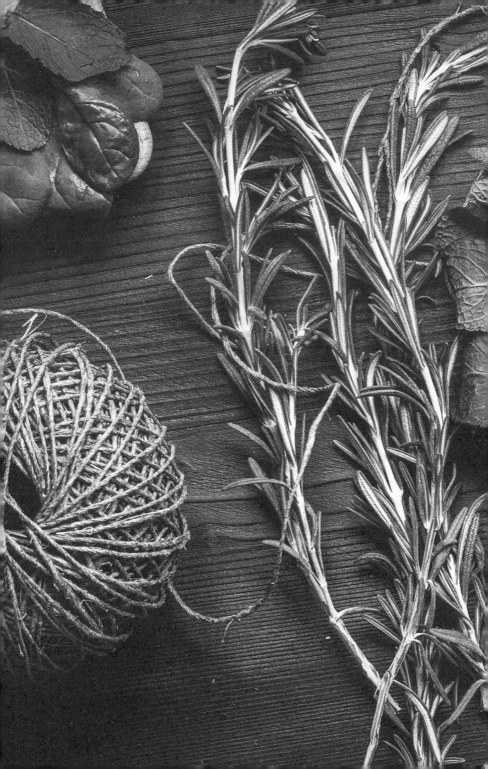

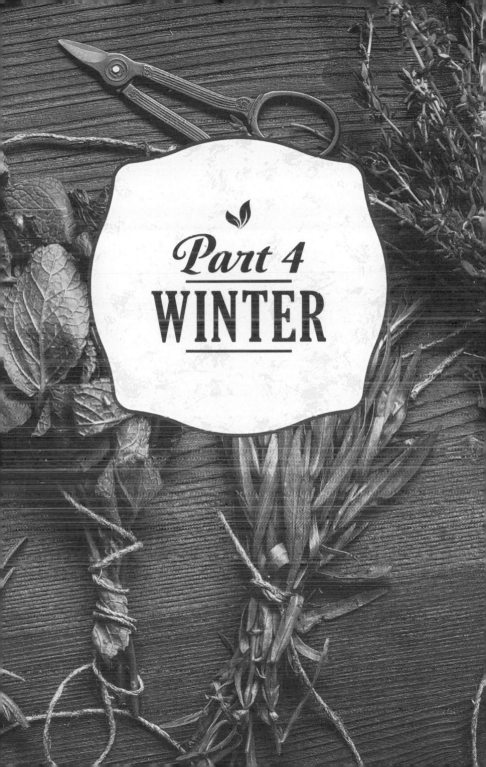

Part 4
WINTER

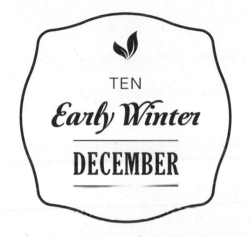

TEN

Early Winter

DECEMBER

It may not be everyone's favorite season, but winter is very important. It is the time to shutter in and think about the year to come. We must have time to regroup and reflect on life and how we have handled it in the past year. It is time for reflection on all the blessings we have been given in the past months.

The winter solstice, which is the shortest day of the year, soon approaches. It is a time of darkness. As we prepare to hibernate, we can look to our health. How are we doing? Have we been keeping up with a good diet? Have we been active? Do we sense changes in our bodies or anything that we might be concerned about? How can we improve?

At this time, we may notice various issues that pop up. These can include indigestion, high blood pressure, goiters, rheumatism, intestinal problems, and liver issues.

As we enter winter, we should have a well-stocked pantry of herbs and roots after the fall harvest. Check what you need to stock up on and get things ready so you will have the ingredients needed to make your recipes.

The vegetables and fruits that can help during this time of year are cauliflower, broccoli, oats, barley, Jerusalem artichokes, kelp, garlic, ginger, carrots, sprouts, apples, raisins, figs, and prunes.

Herbs for Early Winter

Here are the herbs I've categorized as healing for early winter:

cinquefoil (*Potentilla reptans*)

coltsfoot (*Tussilago farfara*); avoid if you have liver issues.

comfrey (*Symphytum officinale*); do not ingest.

fennel (*Foeniculum vulgare*)

horsetail (*Equisetum hyemale*); do not use if taking lithium.

sage (*Salvia officinalis*); do not use if pregnant or breastfeeding.

shepherd's purse (*Capsella bursa-pastoris*)

skullcap (*Scutellaria lateriflora*); do not use if pregnant or breastfeeding.

slippery elm (*Ulmus rubra*)

thyme (*Thymus vulgaris*)

Liver Remedies

Our liver is an important organ, and we should take preventive steps to keep it healthy. Tonics can do that nicely. The immune system is truly the guardian of the whole system. If we can keep the immune system strong, we can better heal ourselves and stay strong.

Liver Tonic

Mix together ½ cup each of chopped red clover and watercress. Pour 1 cup of boiling water over the herbs and cover. Steep 15 minutes. Strain and sweeten with honey. Drink daily for 1 week as a tonic.

Costmary Tea

Costmary tea makes a great tonic for a sluggish liver. Add a small handful of chopped costmary to 1 pint of boiling water. Cover and steep 15 minutes. Strain and drink several cups daily for 1 week as a tonic.

Goldenseal Tonic

Goldenseal, best known as yellowroot, has long been held in high regard as a liver tonic. You can purchase the herb in powdered form and fill your own #00 capsules. Suggested dose is 2 capsules daily for 1 month.

The root can be made into a tea and taken as a tonic for the whole system. Place 1 teaspoon of the chopped root in 1 cup of boiling water, cover, and steep for 15–20 minutes. Strain and drink 1 cup daily for 1 month as a liver tonic or gall bladder treatment. Do not use if pregnant or breastfeeding.

Milk Thistle Treatment

Milk thistle cleans and detoxifies the liver. Purchase the herb in powered form and fill #00 capsules. Dosage is to take 2 capsules twice daily for 1 month.

Sassafras Tonic

This sassafras tonic has been around for many centuries, adds many vitamins and minerals to the system, and is a good all-around tonic at any time of year. It does thin the blood, so take caution if you are anemic or prone to falling. Add 1 teaspoons of sassafras root or bark to 1 cup of boiling water. Cover and steep for 10 minutes. Strain and sweeten with honey. Drink 1 cup as a tonic per season.

Chicory Tonic

Mix together 1 tablespoon each of chicory root, dandelion root, crushed caraway seeds, and ginger root. Simmer gently in 2 cups of water until reduced to half. Strain and add ½ cup of sugar to the liquid and gently boil for 2 minutes. Place the liquid in a sterile jar and refrigerate. To take, add 1 tablespoon of the liquid to 1 cup of boiling water, or add 1 tablespoon to your fruit juice. Drink several times daily for a week as a good tonic.

Beet Tonic

Beets are rich in antioxidants and nutrients such as folate and iron. They clean the blood and stimulate and clean the liver. Eat beets on a regular basis or drink beet juice at least once a week. You can also add the juice to your smoothie mixtures.

To make one serving of a beet smoothie, place 1 large beet, peeled and chopped; 1 apple, cored and chopped; 1 inch of ginger root; the zest of 1 lemon; and 1 cup of water in a blender. Blend until smooth, strain well, and serve over ice.

Cleansing Tea

Simmer 2 cups of chopped honeysuckle leaves and flowers, ½ cup of hawthorn berries, and ½ cup of chopped dandelion root in 1 quart of water for about 15 minutes. Strain and drink 2 cups daily, 1 cup before lunch and 1 cup before dinner, for about 1 week as a tonic. Do not use if taking heart medication.

High Blood Pressure Remedy

The winter season has a tendency to play havoc with us stress wise. The holidays and all the traveling, planning, and massive meal making that come with them can make us frantic. High blood pressure is very common. Many conditions cause it, but stress is a big factor. If we learn to slow down and control stress, we can reduce blood pressure greatly. Meditation is an easy way to get in touch with yourself, and it helps dissipate stress so well. Along with taking a more active role in stress reduction, we can use the following recipe as a natural way to lower our blood pressure. Keep your physician informed of what you are doing.

Primrose Tea

Add 1 teaspoon of primrose to 1 cup of boiling water. Add ½ teaspoon of powdered ginger root. Steep for 10 minutes. This tea can lower high blood pressure if taken daily.

Digestive Remedies

Suffering from indigestion? It is hard not to experience it during winter because we tend to overeat and have the holidays to contend with. Try never to eat when under strain or stress. Drink a natural tea that will help settle the stomach and relieve digestive problems with the following recipes.

Seed Treatment

Most seed herbs can be used to treat digestion problems. Caraway, coriander, fennel, and dill are just a few. Always crush the seeds with a mortar and pestle or grind lightly in a blender. That way you get the full value from the herb.

To make a natural tea, mix together 1 tablespoon each of fennel, aniseed, and dill seeds. Add 1 tablespoon of peppermint or spearmint leaves. Store in a tightly closed container. Place 1 teaspoon of the mixture in 1 cup of boiling water. Cover and steep 15 minutes. Strain and sweeten with honey. Drink after meals to help settle digestive upsets.

Digestion Tea

This recipe can be used as a nervine, tonic, and digestive aid, as well as a remedy for colds and headaches and a way to relax. Using equal amounts of each ingredient, mix together dried skullcap, mullein, chamomile, goldenseal, hyssop, aniseed, and violet leaves. Store in a tightly closed container. Place 1 teaspoon of this mixture in 1 cup of boiling water. Cover and steep 15 minutes. Strain and sweeten with honey. Drink warm before bed for a good night's sleep. Do not use if pregnant or breastfeeding.

Marshmallow Digestive

This tea is especially good to treat digestive problems, colds, and flu. Add ¼ ounce of ginger root and ¼ ounce of willow bark to 1 quart of water. Simmer slowly for about 15 minutes. Add ½ ounce of marshmallow leaves and ¼ ounce of peppermint leaves. Cover and remove from heat. Steep for 20 minutes. Strain and stir in 1 cup of honey. Refrigerate. The dose is 2 tablespoons to 1 cup of warm water as needed for indigestion. This remedy will keep you from feeling nauseous when suffering from the flu or colds, and it soothes the throat. The willow will reduce fever or pain.

Parsley Tea

This recipe treats digestive problems. It acts as a diuretic as well. Add 1 teaspoon each of parsley, yarrow, and chamomile to 2 cups of boiling water. Cover and steep 15 minutes. Strain and sweeten with honey. Drink warm to help settle stomach upsets.

Sea Kelp Aid

If you have a tendency to have low iodine or suffer from goiters, use this remedy; it serves two purposes. It gets iodine in the system and uses kelp to help settle a nervous stomach. Add ½ ounce of powdered sea kelp to 2 cups of boiling water. Cover and steep 15 minutes. Drink as needed for indigestion.

Calming Tea

This tea helps calm a nervous stomach, and it also helps alleviate a nervous headache. Pour 1 cup of boiling water over several sprigs of marjoram and 1 teaspoon of spearmint. Cover and steep 10 minutes. Strain and sweeten with honey if desired. Drink as needed for headaches and indigestion.

Ulcer Treatment

Ulcers can be caused by an excess of acid in the stomach. Neutralizing the acid can soothe the ulcer and help the liver to heal. As funny as it sounds, cayenne pepper is one of the better treatments to help heal ulcers. Place 1 teaspoon of cayenne pepper in 1 cup of hot water. Drink daily as a treatment. It cleans the blood and improves blood circulation.

Red Clover Treatment

Red clover tea is a great way to relieve pain from an ulcer. Add 2 tablespoons of red clover blossoms and 1 teaspoon of lemon balm to 1 cup of boiling water. Cover and steep 15 minutes. Strain and sweeten with honey if desired. Drink 1 cup before meals and before bedtime.

Yogurt Treatment

Eating yogurt on a daily basis helps to treat, heal, and prevent ulcers. Yogurt helps destroy harmful bacteria that causes the formation of acids in the stomach. Eating fruit or berries in the yogurt helps to make it more enjoyable and adds health benefits.

For a tummy-soothing smoothie, put 6 ounces plain regular or Greek yogurt, 1 cup milk or milk alternative of your preference, 6–8 mint leaves or 2–3 drops peppermint essential oil, ½ teaspoon vanilla, and 3–4 ice cubes in a blender. Blend well and enjoy.

Sedative Remedies

There may be times in your life when you need a stronger sedative-type herbal remedy to relieve anxiety symptoms. There are several good herbs to use. Here are some home remedies that use those herbs to make calming teas and capsules.

Primrose Tea

Primrose tea is a great reliever of depression and headaches, and it acts as a sedative. Add 3 teaspoons of dried primrose leaves and flowers to 2 cups of boiling water. Cover and steep 15 minutes. Strain and sweeten with honey. Drink warm as needed.

Skullcap Blend Tea

This blend is great to help relieve tension headaches and to induce sleep. Mix together 1 tablespoon each of skullcap, corn flowers, sage, and chamomile. Store in a tightly closed container. Stir 1 teaspoon of the mixture into 1 cup of boiling water. Cover and steep 10 minutes. Strain and sweeten with honey. Drink as needed. Do not use if pregnant or breastfeeding.

Valerian Capsules

Valerian is a favorite of mine, and valerian capsules make excellent remedies. Using the powdered form of each ingredient, mix 1 tablespoon each of valerian, violets, apple pectin, and sage. The apple pectin is used because it is a blood cleanser. The sage and violets are both sedatives, and the violets add vitamin A to the system. The body needs extra vitamin A during times of stress. Mix the powdered herbs thoroughly, place in #00 capsules, and take 2 capsules every 2 hours as needed. Do not use if pregnant or breastfeeding.

Lavender Headache Capsules

Mix together powdered lavender, catnip, and skullcap. Place in #00 capsules and take 2 as needed. This remedy is good for headaches caused by nervous tension and strain. Do not use if pregnant or breastfeeding.

Pain Remedies

Aches, pains, and arthritis seem worse in cold weather. Thankfully there are many ways to deal with pain, rheumatism, and arthritis using natural methods. Massage is a good way to relieve pain, as well as taking capsules of willow. If you are unable to get powdered willow bark, you can use yarrow or any of the sedative herbs. Yarrow has similar properties to willow and acts as a pain reliever, but I suggest adding at least two other herbs to yarrow capsules. Do research to find herbs that will help with your particular symptoms.

Blended Pain Control

Mix together 1 tablespoon each of powdered buckthorn bark, alfalfa, yarrow, parsley, cayenne pepper, and yucca root. Fill #00 capsules and take 2 daily for 1 week. After the first week, take 3 daily to help control pain. After the second week, take 4 daily.

Ginger Pain Relief

Taking ginger capsules on a daily basis helps with the pain and swelling of rheumatic joints. Simply place powdered ginger in #00 capsules and take 2 daily for as long as you like.

Apple Cider Poultice

Mix equal parts apple cider and water. Heat the mix and apply with a clean cloth to joints. This will help with arthritis pain and swelling.

Comfrey Poultice

Comfrey has pain-relieving properties and makes a great poultice. Place a handful of comfrey leaves in hot water or witch hazel. After the leaves have wilted, place them in a cloth that has been dipped into the comfrey liquid. Apply to the swollen area and keep warm.

Menthol Rub Cream

This is a quick and easy cream to make that can be used as a rub for arthritic conditions. Add 2 tablespoons of menthol crystals to 6 ounces of witch hazel. Add 4 teaspoons of lanolin to the liquid and gently heat in a double boiler until the crystals and lanolin are melted. Remove from heat, pour into tins or jelly jars, and let cool.

Horseradish Poultice

This poultice works well for arthritic pain and sprains. Grate a fresh horseradish root into a small porous bag or cloth and apply to the affected area so the juice can ooze out.

Pain Relief Bath Soak

Mix equal amounts of Epsom salts, sea or table salt, and baking soda in your bathwater. Add up to 10 drops of essential oil(s) of your choice for extra healing. Rosemary is great for sore muscles from overuse or arthritis, and lavender helps relax and ease pain. Take a good, long soak—at least 20 minutes.

Pain Relief Tea

Place 1 teaspoon of dried parsley in 1 cup of boiling water. Add 1 teaspoon of ground ginger and drink daily.

Arthritis Treatment

This tea is another good arthritis remedy. Stir 1 ounce each of honey and apple cider vinegar into 14 ounces of water. Drink daily to alleviate arthritis and rheumatism pain. Lessening pain symptoms will be evident after taking daily for about 1 month.

Brewer's Yeast Treatment

Place 2 tablespoons of brewer's yeast in your morning juice or milk for daily consumption. This helps chronic pain.

Yarrow Poultice

Carefully add several large handfuls of white yarrow to 1 quart of boiling water mixed with 1 pint of apple cider vinegar. Cover and steep 20 minutes. Dip a cloth into the liquid mixture and place the wilted yarrow in the cloth. Fold up the cloth and place it on the affected joint. Place a plastic cover over the pack (plastic wrap works well). Apply a heating pad to keep the pack warm.

ELEVEN
Midwinter

JANUARY

Midwinter is often seen as the starting place of the earth's renewal power. We must respect the powers of tradition and rituals. We have the knowledge of the healing powers of plants and herbs that were discovered by and handed down to us from our elders and ancestors.

Problems with corns, warts, or other topical skin problems are more easily addressed in winter months, as we have less sun exposure. We also have to watch for joint disorders. Extra calcium should be included in your daily diet this time of year.

Foods to focus on during midwinter are spinach, asparagus, cucumbers, lettuce, almonds, lentils, brown beans, whole wheat, rye, barley, fish, milk, strawberries, figs, plums, blueberries, and coconuts.

Herbs for Midwinter

The following is a list of herbs I've categorized as especially healing for midwinter:

apple (*Pyrus malus*)

burdock (*Arctium lappa*)

butcher's-broom (*Ruscus aculeatus*)

chamomile (*Anthemis nobilis, Matricaria chamomilla*)

chickweed (*Stellaria media*)

eyebright (*Euphrasia officinalis*)

honeysuckle (*Diervilla lonicera*)

Irish moss (*Chondrus crispus, Gigartina mamillosa*)

lavender (*Lavandula angustifolia*)

lemongrass (*Cymbopogon citratus*)

mullein (*Verbascum thapsus*)

pansy (*Viola tricolor*)

parsley (*Petroselinum crispum*)

sheep's sorrel (*Rumex acetosella*); use in low doses only.

sweet woodruff (*Galium odoratum*)

valerian (*Valeriana officinalis*); avoid if you have stomach or heart issues.

Cleansing Tonics

Cleansing tonics help strengthen the whole body and help the immune system balance and work as it should. They also contain many vitamins and minerals the body needs. At least once per year, try using a whole-body tonic to boost the system.

Sheep's Sorrel Tonic

Sheep's sorrel serves to internally cleanse the whole system. Many use it as a whole-body tonic. It strengthens the immune system and is used for skin disorders and eruptions, such as boils. It will also help alleviate fever and inflammatory disorders. Carefully place 1 large handful of sheep's sorrel in 1 pint of boiling water. Cover and steep for 15 minutes. Strain and drink a small amount daily for 1 week if using for a specific healing purpose. This is a good tea to drink 1 week out of every month.

Chickweed Tea

Chickweed contains many vitamins and minerals. The plant can be used in salads, as a cooked side dish, or as a tea. It is an inexpensive, delicious addition to our diet that has been there for the taking all along. Chickweed acts as a tonic for the whole body and cleanses impurities in the blood. It is one of the best ways to protect the skin from various disorders.

Chop up several tablespoons of chickweed and pour 1 cup of boiling water over the herb. Cover and steep 15 minutes. Strain and drink several times daily for as long as you feel it necessary.

Jude's Tincture

This tincture serves many purposes and is helpful in fighting colds and flu. It can be used externally to clean wounds and treat skin disorders.

To make this tincture, mash 1 ounce of garlic and pour 1 pint of alcohol over the herb. Use either vodka or brandy. Add 1 ounce of dried white yarrow, ¼ ounce of echinacea root, and 1 ounce of nasturtium leaves or flowers. Cover and keep in a warm, sunny spot for 2 weeks. Shake or stir daily. After 2 weeks, strain out the herbs and store the liquid in a dark place.

The yarrow acts as a pain reliever, garlic is a natural antibiotic, nasturtium helps clear mucus from the system, and echinacea is a blood purifier, lymphatic cleanser, and antibiotic. Dosage is ½ dropper as needed. Mix the dosage into juice or stir into hot water to drink as a tea.

Skin Care Remedies

Our skin absorbs chemicals from the atmosphere and beauty products. Not using commercial soaps can be very beneficial. Making your own health care products is a natural way to start taking responsibility for your own health. Using hand lotions, creams, and rinses made at home saves a lot of money and is a healthy alternative.

Healing Body Lotion

Place 1 cup of olive oil in a stainless steel pan along with 2 tablespoons of lanolin and ¼ ounce beeswax. Add 1 tablespoon of cold-pressed castor oil if you are prone to warts. Heat slightly, just enough to melt all ingredients, and add ½ cup almond oil. Mix in about 25 drops of essential oils that are especially healing for the skin, such as lavender, rose, rose geranium, and chamomile. Add the oil from several broken vitamin E capsules. The vitamin E helps heal the skin. It also acts as a preservative in some measure. Stir continuously while cooling until the desired consistency is reached. Store in a tightly closed container. Use daily as a skin cream.

Shepherd's Purse Skin Salve

Many consider shepherd's purse to be a pest, but it has long been held in high regard by those aware of its amazing qualities. It was used as a hemostat during World War I when other herbs were unavailable. A salve made from the herb can be used to treat wounds, ulcers, injuries, and skin disorders of all kinds.

Place several handfuls of the herb and 1 pint of unsalted lard in a pot. Simmer very slowly for 30 minutes. Remove from heat and strain. Break about 4 vitamin E capsules into the mixture. Stir thoroughly, place in sterile containers, and use as needed for cuts, scrapes, rashes, and wounds.

Dry Skin Moisturizer

The ingredients we need to make natural remedies are usually as close to us as our refrigerator or kitchen cabinet. A little mixing and we have a stocked natural-health pantry! To make a moisturizer for dry skin, mix 1 egg yolk with 1 tablespoon of glycerin. Smooth on face, leave on for 5 minutes, and rinse thoroughly.

Skin Renewal Tonic

This skin-renewing remedy can be used to help rejuvenate skin that has been previously overexposed to the sun. We need to be exposed to sunlight in a limited manner in order for our bodies to be able to make vitamin D. Without this important vitamin, we may suffer from bone deficiencies. During winter, we don't receive all we need from the sun because of the shortened days and cloud-covered, gray days. Mix ½ cup each of lemon juice, glycerin, and rose water. Shake well and apply to the body after your bath. The zinc helps repair damaged cells, and the vitamin C helps us absorb and utilize vitamin D.

Skin Conditioner

This tonic helps prevent boils and other skin conditions by cleansing the blood. Place 1 ounce each of burdock root, thyme, dock, violet leaves, and sage in 1 quart of water. Boil until liquid is halved. Strain and drink ½ cup daily for 1 week. Do not use if pregnant or breastfeeding.

Parsley Face Tonic

Parsley makes a good tea thanks to its diuretic properties, but it's also great for external help. Place a large handful of chopped parsley in a bowl and pour 1 cup of boiling water over the herb. Cover and steep 30 minutes. Strain the liquid, dip a clean cloth into the parsley liquid, and apply to the face as a compress for 15 minutes, dipping the cloth back into the warm liquid as it cools.

Burdock Acne Treatment

Burdock is another herb that can serve in several ways. It is a great astringent and good for treating oily skin. Place 2 handfuls of burdock root and 2 cups of water in a pan. Bring to a boil and reduce heat to a simmer. Cover and simmer for 15 minutes. Strain and dip a clean cloth into the burdock liquid. Apply as a compress to the face daily to combat acne and oily skin.

Thyme Astringent

Thyme is an astringent and will unclog pores and help treat acne. Place 3 tablespoons of thyme into a bowl and pour 1 cup of boiling water over the herb. Cover and steep 15 minutes. Use daily as a rinse to treat acne or oily skin.

Strawberry Acne Treatment

Strawberries can be used externally as a treatment for acne or other skin disorders. Simply crush a strawberry and rub it over the face. Leave it on the skin for 15 minutes before rinsing off.

Coltsfoot Toner

Coltsfoot makes a great toner to use after cleansing the skin to clean the pores. It softens and soothes the skin and helps minimize wrinkles. Pour ½ cup of boiling water over 2 tablespoons each of dried coltsfoot leaves, fennel seeds, and dried lemongrass. Cover and steep 15 minutes. Strain and add ½ cup plain yogurt and a small handful of oatmeal to the liquid. After washing the face, place a warm cloth over the face for a few minutes. Remove the cloth and spread the warm herbal mixture on the face. Relax and leave on the skin for at least 10 minutes. Add a little lemon juice to the rinse water and rinse the face thoroughly.

Diuretic Remedies

It is important to keep the urinary tract and bowels open and clear because they affect the skin, and prevention is better than trying to cure after the fact. There are ways you can keep regular through your daily diet. Eat plenty of foods high in fiber and drink plenty of water daily. Drinking water also helps flush the kidneys and bladder and helps keep pores open.

Corn Silk Tea

Corn silk tea is a great way to treat any problems of the urinary tract. Add several tablespoons of dried corn silk to 1 cup of boiling water. Cover and steep 15 minutes. Strain and drink several times a day for 2 days. This is a strong diuretic so do not continue the treatment for more than 2 days.

Parsley Tea

To prepare a parsley tea to use as a urinary tract cleanser, pour 1 cup of boiling water over 2 tablespoons of chopped parsley. If using dried parsley, use 1 tablespoon. Cover and steep 15 minutes. Drink several times a day for 3 days.

Lemon Thyme Cleanser

Thyme is an astringent and has antiseptic properties that clean the urinary system. Lemon thyme makes a pleasant tea. Chop 1 tablespoon of lemon thyme and add to 1 cup of boiling water. Cover and steep 15 minutes. Strain and drink daily for 1 week. Sweeten with apple pectin if desired.

Burdock Tonic

Burdock is a great blood purifier and diuretic, and this burdock tonic is very helpful. Place 1 ounce each of burdock root, dandelion root, and sassafras bark in 1 quart of water. Boil until the liquid is reduced by half. Strain and add ¼ cup of the herbal liquid to 1 cup of hot water. Keep the rest of the mixture refrigerated in a sealed container. Sweeten with honey and drink several cups a day for 2 weeks, making more as needed.

Clove Laxative

A common spice in your kitchen cabinet can be used as a natural method for treating constipation. Place 1 tablespoon of whole cloves in a cup. Pour 1 cup of boiling water over the cloves. Cover and steep overnight. Strain and drink the following morning.

Cinquefoil Tea

Cinquefoil tea has many uses. It is a good blood cleanser that can help stop diarrhea and other bowel complaints. It can stop the bleeding of the gums if used as a gargle, and it can be used externally for healing sores and ulcers. To make the tea to use as a gargle, add 1 teaspoon of cinquefoil to 1 cup boiling water. Cover and steep 15 minutes. To make the tea to treat sores and ulcers, add 1 tablespoon of cinquefoil to 1 cup of boiling water and steep until cool. To help stop diarrhea, steep 1 tablespoon in 1 cup of boiling water and sip throughout the day. Use as an external wash for open ulcers, wounds, and sores.

Mood-Lifting Remedies

With winter comes less sunlight and vitamin D3, a decrease in activity and interaction with others, and a disruption of melatonin levels that can affect sleep and mood, which can all make us more prone to depression. Thankfully many herbs can help with a depressed mood. Chamomile, peppermint, lemon balm, and lavender are just a few.

Pansy Tea

Add several teaspoons of chopped pansy leaves and flowers to 1 cup of boiling water. Cover and steep for 15 minutes. Strain and sweeten with honey if desired.

Sage Tea

Sage tea is a relaxant as well as a good headache remedy. Add several different herbs for flavor if desired. Sage added to apple tea is a good treatment for the blood as well as a light relaxant.

Pour 1 cup of boiling water over 1 teaspoon of dried sage leaves. Steep 8–10 minutes. Add a dried apple slice and sweeten to taste. Do not use if pregnant or breastfeeding.

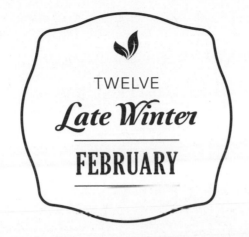

TWELVE
Late Winter
FEBRUARY

There is a light at the end of the tunnel. Spring is not far off. We've made it to the end of winter and the promise of future life is awaiting us under the cold. The cold ground is like a secret present waiting to be opened. We've been huddled by the hearth of the home for quite some time. It makes sense to keep cleansing so we will be ready for all the action soon to come. We also need to make sure our feet are in good shape so that we can be the best we can be when warm weather comes.

A Note about Sodium and Iron

The minerals we should focus on are salt and iron. Salt's mission is to unite with the water within us and make it useful. There must be a balance, or your legs and ankles will swell. Natural diuretics help flush out stored water. Iron strengthens the immune system and helps the blood receive oxygen, which helps the circulatory system keep moving.

Foods to maintain good sodium and iron levels during this time include spinach, cabbage, cauliflower, brussels sprouts, asparagus, lettuce, radish, lentils, cucumber, carrots, chestnuts, apple, figs, strawberries, coconuts, peas, beans, onions, rice, potatoes, turnips, milk and milk products, wheat, rye, eggs, cherries, and pears.

Herbs for Late Winter

Here are the herbs that I've categorized as especially healing for late winter:

apple (*Pyrus malus*)

calendula (*Calendula officinalis*)

cherry (*Prunus avium*)

comfrey (*Symphytum officinale*); do not ingest.

dandelion (*Taraxacum officinale*)

dock (*Rumex* spp.)

fenugreek (*Trigonella foenum-graecum*)

feverfew (*Chrysanthemum parthenium*)

ginger (*Zingiber officinale*)

goldenseal (*Hydrastis canadensis*)

Irish moss (*Chondrus crispus, Gigartina mamillosa*)

kelp (*Fucus vesiculosus*)

lavender (*Lavandula angustifolia*)

lemon balm (*Melissa officinalis*)

oak gall (*Quercus infectoria*)

pansy (*Viola tricolor*)

parsley (*Petroselinum crispum*)

plantain (*Plantago major*)

prickly lettuce (*Lactuca virosa, L. serriola*)

sage (*Salvia officinalis*); do not use if pregnant or breastfeeding.

sassafras (*Sassafras albidum*)

thyme (*Thymus vulgaris*)

valerian (*Valeriana officinalis*); avoid if you have stomach or
heart issues.

violet (*Viola odorata*)

wild strawberry (*Fragaria virginiana*) and garden strawberry
(*Fragaria vesca*)

Restorative Tonics

Tonics can help add needed minerals to your system. However, you
should be careful not to overload the body, so pay attention to dosage requirements.

Ginger Tea

Ginger acts as a stimulant and a diuretic to flush the kidneys. Adding
some to your daily tea is a good habit, as is making a tea from ginger
root by itself. Add 1 teaspoon of freshly ground ginger to 1 cup of
boiling water. Cover and steep 15 minutes. Strain and sweeten with
honey if desired. Drink daily.

Plantain Tea

By observing wildlife, we can find better herbs for
us to use. This is true of plantain. Rabbits love
it! Plantain has long been considered a weed
that needs to be removed from lawns, but
it makes a great diuretic as a tea and is
often taken as a tonic.

Place several fresh leaves or 1 tablespoon
of the dried herb in 1 cup of boiling water. Cover
and steep for 15 minutes. Strain and drink several times

daily for 1 week as a tonic. Increase the amount of the herb used if you are taking it as a diuretic.

Celery Seed Tea

A good addition to any spice cabinet is celery seed. It makes a great diuretic tea. Add 1 teaspoon of celery seeds to 1 cup of boiling water. Cover and steep for 15 minutes. Strain and drink several cups daily for 2–3 days to clean the urinary system.

Foot Remedies and Treatments

When treating the body for disease, many people overlook the importance of foot care. The feet carry the weight of the body and are important to our general health.

Foot problems come in many guises, including cuts, corns, and other skin disorders. You might encounter boils, skin ulcers, and bunions. Gout is caused by too much uric acid in the system, and tonics that act as diuretics are very helpful.

The following remedies can treat several different disorders—or simply be a treat for the feet. A long soak in a footbath does much to relieve symptoms of tiredness and can revive your cheerful attitude!

Lavender Footbath

Lavender tea is soothing to drink, and adding some lavender to a footbath is very relaxing. To make the tea, add 1 teaspoon of lavender to 1 cup of boiling water. Cover and steep 15 minutes. Drink while soaking the feet. For the footbath, add 4 tablespoons of the herb to 1 cup of boiling water, then cover and steep 20 minutes. Strain and add to the footbath water.

Lemon Balm Soak

Lemon balm serves two functions. It makes a good footbath, and a poultice made from the tea dispels bunions and corns. To treat a bunion, make a strong tea using 4–5 tablespoons of lemon balm and 1 cup of boiling water. Cover and steep until cool. Dip a small piece of bread in the tea and apply to the bunion. Bandage and leave on overnight. Repeat until improvement is evident.

Toenail Helper

To soften the area around the toenails and strengthen the nails, mix together 3 tablespoons each of raw linseed oil, honey, and almond oil. Massage each nail and the surrounding area. This treatment is also good to strengthen the fingernails. Keep the toenails trimmed straight across to prevent problems with hangnails or ingrown nails.

St. John's Wort Tincture

St. John's wort makes a great pain reliever for cuts and wounds. It is also at the top of the list when it comes to bacteria killers. Having a tincture made from St. John's wort on hand and ready to use is a good preventive measure and the sign of a well-stocked home medicine cabinet.

To make the tincture, place whatever amount of St. John's wort you have into a jar and cover the herb with vodka or brandy. Cap tightly and place in a warm, sunny area for 2 weeks. Strain, pour into a sterile container, and label.

You can also prepare the tincture using olive oil. To make it with oil, place the flowers and leaves in a jar of olive oil and let sit in a warm, sunny spot for 6–8 weeks. Strain and store in a dark cupboard. This is a great pain reliever, especially for nerve pain.

From the oil, you can make a salve by adding beeswax and honey or vitamin E oil to preserve the mixture. To make the salve, take ⅔ cup of the strained oil, 1 tablespoon plus 1 teaspoon of melted beeswax, and 6 drops of vitamin E oil and mix well. Pour into small jars or tins with wide openings and let cool. The salve should be firm to the touch but spreadable.

Any of these forms of the recipe can be used to treat corns, calluses, and any skin fungus like athlete's foot. It helps tremendously with pain, reduces itching, and helps heal burns with no or minimal scarring.

Silver Birchbark Footbath

For those aching feet with arthritis, there is nothing better than to make a footbath using 4–5 handfuls of silver birchbark to 1 quart of boiling water. Cover and steep for 30 minutes. Strain out the birchbark and use the liquid as a footbath for a relaxing soak.

Calendula and Mint Footbath

Any of the mint herbs are good to add to your footbath. They are stimulating and help take away that tired feeling. Adding calendula to the water helps heal any skin disorders and is relaxing. Add 2 tablespoons of calendula and/or mint to 1 cup of boiling water. Cover and steep until cool. Strain out the herbs and use the liquid as a footbath.

Corn Treatments

Corns can be very painful. There are several ways to treat them, but it is best to avoid them by using the preventive measure of taking good care of your feet. Let the feet breathe by going barefoot as much as possible. I go barefoot most of the time indoors and out. This allows my feet to touch Mother Earth and helps me feel connected to her.

When you do wear shoes, they should fit well and be very comfortable. Money spent on good shoes is well spent—simply because we spend so much time on our feet.

Onion Corn Treatment

Onions are very useful when it comes to healing corns. Before you go to bed, slice an onion and place a piece on the corn. Bandage the area and leave it on overnight. This treatment takes several weeks, but it does work. Garlic is a good substitute if onions are not available.

Vinegar Poultice

Bruise a small amount of ivy leaves, cover the leaves with apple cider vinegar, and let them sit overnight. Strain out the leaves. Dip a small piece of bread in the mixture and apply it to the corn. Bandage and leave on during the day if possible. Repeat the process at night. Continue until the corn disappears. The wet bread molds to the corn and holds the liquid to the area that needs help. Bread can be used to apply a poultice in any area that may be difficult to treat. It stays in place and allows the spot to receive the full effect of treatment.

Athlete's Foot Treatments

Athlete's foot is caused by a fungal infection of the outer layer of dead skin on the feet. If feet are allowed to breathe properly, the problem will not exist. The cold winds blow this time of season, and we can't help but bundle up with thick socks and boots or shoes. This can cause sweat, though, and the cold rain or snow can also leave our feet moist. Don't allow the feet to stay damp. Dampness creates many infections and disorders. Take your shoes off at home to help your feet stay healthy. Many of the herbs mentioned in this section are considered astringent in nature and can help dispel many problems if we use them as a foot wash.

Thyme Treatment

Thyme helps rid the skin of infectious germs. Place 2 tablespoons of thyme in 1 cup of boiling water. Cover and steep until cool. Strain and add to a footbath as a treatment or use as a rinse.

Apple Cider Vinegar Foot Treatment

Soak a cloth in apple cider vinegar and apply to the feet. Do not rinse. Dip cotton balls in vinegar and place between the toes. Put socks on and leave on overnight.

Red Clover Rinse

Place 2 tablespoons of red clover in ½ cup of boiling water. Cover and steep until cool. Strain and mix with enough cornstarch to make a paste. Apply all over the feet, put socks on, and leave on overnight. Rinse feet using the thyme treatment in the morning.

Lemon Juice Astringent

Lemon juice can be very helpful when treating athlete's foot. Apply plenty of lemon juice to the feet and do not rinse off. Allow the juice to dry naturally on the feet. Reapply the juice several times daily and before bed.

Valerian Treatment

Valerian tincture is a good healer for athlete's foot. Place 2 table-spoons of valerian in 1 cup of boiling water. Cover and steep until cool. Strain and dip a cotton ball into the herbal liquid and apply all over the feet. Allow to dry and do not rinse off.

This tincture also helps treat ulcers and sores. Apply it to the area with a clean cotton ball frequently.

Leg Treatments

Swelling in the calf or leg can be caused by serious medical conditions, and a physician must be consulted. Bed rest is important, as well as keeping the limb immobile.

Butcher's-Broom Treatment

Butcher's-broom helps prevent blood clots from forming and is great for general inflammation. Make a tea by adding 1 tablespoon of butcher's-broom root to 1 cup of boiling water. Steep 10 minutes, strain, and add sweetener if desired. This tea isn't for everyone, as some people can experience headaches or nausea as a side effect, so use care.

If you have problems with phlebitis, it can be helpful to take butcher's-broom on a daily basis. Mix together 1 tablespoon each of butcher's-broom, apple pectin, cayenne pepper, and lecithin. Place in #00 capsules and take 2 daily. This treatment will remove toxins from the body, prevent blood clots, and help with circulation.

Cayenne Pepper Tea

Cayenne pepper is helpful if you have circulatory problems. Add 1 teaspoon of cayenne pepper to 1 cup of hot water. Drink daily as an aid to increase blood circulation.

Leg Ulcer Treatment

There are many ways to treat leg ulcers. One of the best is using calendula flowers as a wash for open ulcers. Place 1 cup of calendula leaves and flowers in 2 cups of boiling water. Cover and steep until cool. Use as a rinse after thoroughly cleaning the open ulcer. Pack the ulcer with powdered sugar and apply a light bandage. Change the bandage frequently and repeat the process of washing, rinsing with the calendula tea, and applying the powdered sugar to the area.

Comfrey Poultice

Place 4 leaves of comfrey into a blender along with ¼ cup of water. Blend well and apply to the ulcer as a poultice daily. After removing the poultice, break 3 capsules of goldenseal oil and apply the oil directly to the ulcer. Leave the ulcer exposed to the open air as often as possible.

Violet Tea Wash

A violet tea wash is an economical, quick, and easy way to treat ulcers and other leg issues. Place a small handful of violet leaves and flowers in 1 cup of boiling water. Cover, steep until cool, and strain. Soak a clean cloth in the herb liquid and apply to the area. Leave it on overnight if you can. Continue until improvement is noticed. Use the tea as a wash after cleaning the wound or ulcer.

Comfrey leaves can be added to the tea to provide even more healing power when it's used as a wash—but only add a few and consult your physician before using. The toxicity of the comfrey plant can be absorbed through the skin. Do **not** drink the tea if comfrey is added. Yarrow can be added for pain relief and more healing properties. Red clover is another great herb to use when treating sores because it helps heal the area quickly.

Boil Treatments

Boils are painful, red pus-filled bumps on the skin caused by infected hair follicles. They happen anywhere on the body, but they most often develop on the groin, face, or neck, or under the arms. If you have one, you will want to use a remedy that draws the poison out and helps with inflammation.

Parsley Boil Treatment

An external treatment for boils is a parsley poultice. Place a small handful of parsley in 1 cup of boiling water. Cover and steep 15 minutes. Strain and fold the parsley into a clean cloth that has been dipped in the parsley liquid. Place the poultice on the boil and wrap with a plastic covering. Place a heating pad over the poultice. Keep the pad on 10–15 minutes at a time 3–4 times a day until it comes to a head.

Pansy Boil Treatment

To treat a boil, cut up a handful of pansies and place them in 1 cup of boiling water. Cover and steep for 15 minutes. Remove the herb from the liquid and place it on the boil. Dip a clean cloth in the liquid and place the cloth on the boil to hold the wilted herb in place. Bandage and leave on overnight.

Linseed Oil Treatment

Apply linseed oil freely to the boil to soften it and aid in healing.

Irish Moss Salve

This salve can be used to treat boils and other skin disorders. Pour ½ cup of boiling water over ¼ ounce of Irish moss and 3 table-spoons each of chopped comfrey and violet leaves. Steep until cool. Remove the herbs and add the oil from 3 broken capsules of vitamin E. Mix well and apply as a salve to the affected area.

Red Clover Boil Treatment

Red clover is a wonderful blood cleanser and purifier. This herb has often been used to clear up boils and skin problems. Add 1 table-spoon of red clover flowers to 1 cup of boiling water. Cover and steep 15 minutes. Strain and sweeten with honey if desired. Drink daily, if possible, to prevent skin disorders.

Gout Treatments

Gout is a type of arthritis where the person accumulates an excess of uric acid in the body, which then accumulates as crystals in the joints, particularly in the foot and big toe.

Cherry Gout Treatment

Cherries are known to help prevent gout attacks if eaten on a daily basis. There are many ways to get cherries in your daily diet. Canning your own will give you access to the juice and fruit. Drink the juice after sweetening, and mix the fruit with yogurt or other fruit. The fruit can also be used in baking.

To make a cherry gout treatment, add 1 pint of cherries to 1 pint of water. Simmer on low heat for 30 minutes. Strain and add 1 pint of honey to the liquid and stir. Refrigerate and take 2 tablespoons daily to prevent a gout attack. One tablespoon also acts as a cough suppressant.

Pear Gout Prevention

Pears are great to help prevent an attack of gout. Eat 3 pears daily to help stop an attack from coming on.

Apple Gout Treatment

Drinking apple tea is another great way to treat gout. Place several slices of dried apple in 1 cup of boiling water, cover, and steep 15 minutes. Remove the apple slices and drink frequently. The apple tea helps remove the uric acid from the system, and excess uric acid is what causes the pain of a gout attack.

Eating apple pectin on a daily basis is another way to prevent gout. You can use apple pectin as a sugar substitute.

Strawberry Gout Treatment

Strawberries are a natural way to help ward off gout attacks. Place 4–6 strawberry leaves in 1 cup of boiling water. Cover and steep for 20 minutes. Strain and sweeten with honey or apple pectin. Drink as often as desired.

Fenugreek Poultice

Place 1 ounce of fenugreek seed in ½ cup of boiling water. Cover and steep until cool. Strain. The resulting liquid can be applied as a poultice to the inflamed area to reduce pain.

Comfrey Poultice

Comfrey is a pain reliever and great for use in a poultice. Put a large handful of comfrey leaves in 1 pint of boiling water. Cover and steep until lukewarm. Remove the wilted leaves and place them in a clean cloth that has been soaked in the liquid. Place the cloth on the affected area. Cover with a heating pad to keep warm. Replace the poultice frequently. Some caution should be used when using comfrey concerning liver toxicity. Do not ingest, and use externally only on those over 4 years old.

Apple Cider Vinegar Poultice

Heat some apple cider vinegar until warm. Dip a cloth into the vinegar and apply as a poultice to the area. Repeat the process, keeping the cloth warm. You can apply a heating pad over the poultice to keep the cloth warm. Wrap the pad with a towel or plastic wrap.

Daily Drink

Add 1 teaspoon each of honey and apple cider vinegar to 1 glass of water and drink daily in the morning. This is of great help with gout, arthritis, and other related conditions.

Craving Remedies

Winter seems to be when we are more tempted to overindulge in alcohol. This is a time full of holiday gatherings, and drinks are often added to the celebrations. Because we are cooped up indoors and dealing with decreased sunlight and gloomy days, a glass or two of wine or spirits seems a good idea, and a little can easily turn into too much. The treatments in this section can help dampen down the desire to drink.

Honey Treatment

Often when we overindulge, it is said to be evidence of a lack of potassium in the body. Honey has potassium, which means it is one way to replace potassium fast. It helps stop the craving for alcohol. Before an individual is sober, give them 2 tablespoons of honey every 20 minutes until they fall asleep. Continue the honey treatment the next day, giving them some every 20 minutes. This natural treatment will also help the individual avoid a nasty hang-over. Do not use this treatment if the individual is diabetic.

Apple Cider Vinegar Treatment

Some people crave a beer after putting in a hard day at work. Beer has a high acid content. This need can be filled by adding apple cider vinegar to the diet on a daily basis.

Cravings, addictions, and a nervous disposition just may point to an imbalance in the body. According to Dr. D. C. Jarvis, a tincture called Lugol's solution should be taken regularly to restore the lack of potassium fast. Lugol's solution is made up of 5 percent elemental iodine dissolved in a 10 percent solution of potassium iodine.

> Because we may live in an iodine-poor area; because drinking water may be treated with chlorine; because we may be sick too often, lack energy and endurance, develop nervous tension, lack the ability of clear thinking, and accumulate unwanted fat … the Lugol's solution is an inexpensive preparation to take.[5]

Adding a drop of this solution to apple cider vinegar, honey, and water on a regular basis will help restore these valuable minerals to the system. But there are herbs that also contain vital minerals.

....
5. Jarvis, *Folk Medicine*, 192.

Yarrow Treatment

This yarrow treatment is a good herbal mixture because yarrow has pain-relieving properties and adds extra potassium to the system. Valerian is added because it is excellent in treating depression and tension. Ginger is added because it settles an upset stomach and stops nausea.

Mix together dried yarrow, valerian, and ginger in equal amounts. Store in a tightly closed container. Add 1 teaspoon of this mixture to 1 cup of boiling water. Cover and steep for 10 minutes. Strain and sweeten with honey. Drink as needed to help prevent alcohol craving and banish depression.

Raspberry Tincture

Add 1 quart of black raspberries to 1 pint of apple cider vinegar. Boil until the liquid is halved. Strain, add 1 pint of honey, and simmer for 30 minutes. Pour into a sterile jar, label, and refrigerate. Take 1 tablespoon as needed to prevent alcohol craving.

Lettuce Tea

This tea can help with cravings. Chop 1 cup of lettuce and pour 1 cup of boiling water over it. Cover and steep for 30 minutes. Strain and drink before bed to promote good sleep.

Liver Cleanse

Alcohol can cause liver damage. Thankfully a tincture made from sweet woodruff is a wonderful liver treatment. It is a good idea to do a liver cleanse once or twice a year at the change of seasons. Cleansing the body can help reduce inflammation, which is a cause of body pain.

Place ½ cup of crushed sweet woodruff into a jar. Pour ½ cup of olive oil over the herb. Allow to sit for 2 weeks in a warm, sunny area. Strain and break several capsules of vitamin E into the oil tincture. Shake well and give ½ a dropperful under the tongue daily as a liver cleanser.

CONCLUSION

As we have discovered, plants and how we can use them for keeping ourselves healthy follow the flow of the seasons. The following quote seems to sum this up perfectly and ties in with my mother's thoughts entirely.

> As I've grown older and learned to recognize the patterns within myself, I've come to understand my body better. Like the tides are inextricably tied to the moon and sunflowers chase the sun, so, too, am I tethered to the natural world. It's an interesting paradigm shift, to take a step back from the modern pressures of life—constant screen time, juggling household tasks, navigating packed calendars—and realize I am not separate from nature: I am part of it—and it is part of me.[6]

It is important that we rediscover the ability to follow along with nature instead of going against it. If you keep your immune system strong, illness will not come knocking at your door nearly as often. When you feel good, your whole outlook is sunny and bright. This is what we all strive for, and it's my wish that we all glide through the seasons healthy and happy. And if we need to, use the wonderful gift of the herbs and plants that surround us to help us accomplish it.

. . . .
6. Kukuk, "Under the Spell of the Seasons."

RECIPE INDEX

Part 1: Spring

Chapter 2: Mid-Spring: April

Part 2: Summer

Chapter 4: Early Summer: June

Part 3: Fall

Chapter 7: Early Fall: September

PREPARATION OF CAPSULES, SALVES, SYRUPS, AND TINCTURES

Preparing salves and liniments for future use is a good idea. It will save you time. If you prepare them in advance, you will have them on hand for emergencies or for everyday use. My daughter keeps a list of frequently used recipes taped inside the door of her herbal cabinet. Of course, there will always be recipes that you simply cannot prepare ahead of time, but their ingredients can be placed in tightly closed containers and clearly labeled. Always use sterile containers and be sure to clearly label each with the contents, use, dosage, and date made.

It may take time to build up a nice supply of the kind of herbs needed for your remedies, but it is well worth the effort. If you are going to have a big supply of herbs, you must have containers in which to store them. I collect antique tin canisters and keep my dried herbs in them. Dark glass bottles are said to be the best kind of storage container, but I love my tins. I mainly use them for storing beeswax, capsules, and other miscellaneous things that I need to prepare herbal remedies. I place my canisters in a large cabinet that has glass doors. It holds a prominent place in my living room. It really does make a nice addition to the room and is very handy.

It is important to put a preservative in the recipes that you plan to store for indefinite periods of time. If honey is used in the recipe, that will be sufficient, as honey is a great preservative. If you are not using honey, adding the oil from several vitamin E capsules to your herbal mixtures is another way to preserve them. Benzoin is called for in some of the recipes included in this book. This is a preservative, and you will not need to add any other preservatives if you are using it.

Preparing Capsules

Herbal remedies may be taken in capsule form as well as by teas or tinctures. Often, capsules are more convenient to take during the day while we are at work, or while away from home for an extended length of time. There are many reasons that you would want to take capsules instead of a tea or tincture. If the treatment you are seeking is long term, such as for high blood pressure, then you would definitely want to try the capsules.

You can purchase empty gelatin capsules at your local health food store or pharmacy. There are many different sizes of capsules, but you probably would use the #00 capsules the most. To fill a capsule, simply take it apart and fill the largest end, replacing the top to close it. The leafy herbs can be powdered in your food processor if necessary, but the root herbs must be purchased in powdered form.

The dosage would be the same as if you were taking an infusion, which is a tea remedy. If the infusion calls for 3 cups a day, then you would take 1 capsule three times a day with water.

Preparing Salves

Salves need a preservative because they are often used for cuts and wounds and as such need to be free from bacteria. A good preservative to use is tincture of benzoin, which you can purchase from your local drugstore. It is inexpensive and is necessary for the preparation of your salves. Choose stainless steel, glass, or earthenware when you are looking for bowls or containers in which to mix or store your herbal preparations. The containers you use to store the mixtures should be airtight and sterile.

It is helpful to know what the basic ingredients of a salve are. The ingredients used to make the salves are the herbs you plan to use, an oil, some beeswax, and the preservative. The best kind of oil to use is olive or sesame. Do not use the drying oils, such as soybean and linseed.

Basic Salve Recipe

To make a basic salve, begin by heating the oil just to boiling (in a stainless steel or glass pan). Add the herbs of your choice and simmer, covered, for about 3 hours. Instead of heating it up on the stove, you can prepare this mixture in the oven if you like. Just keep the temperature low and the container covered.

If part of your herbal recipe includes barks or roots, place these in the oil first and simmer them for the first 1½ hours before adding additional flowers or leaves. If using fresh herbs, always leave the lid off the container for the first 30 minutes in order to allow the water to evaporate from the herbs.

After the mixture is ready, strain and add the beeswax. (You will need about 1½ ounces of beeswax for every 2 cups of oil that you use.) Next, add ½ teaspoon of the tincture of benzoin for every 2 cups of oil used. Mix well. To test for consistency, put a small amount of the salve in a tablespoon and place in the refrigerator. If the salve is not thick enough, add a little more beeswax. When the desired consistency is reached, pour the mixture into labeled jars.

The salve will keep for years. I place mine in small jars so that I have plenty to give family members and friends.

Preparing Syrups

When preparing the cough syrups, the dried herbal mixtures are generally decocted (boiled). The mixture is then strained. Then the honey is added and the mixture is allowed to simmer an additional 30 minutes. Add the flavoring after the mixture has cooled.

There are certain types of herbs that are generally included when preparing cough syrups. They are as follows:

1. *Stimulants or activators:* a stimulant is an agent that temporarily increases functional activity. For example, a diuretic increases the secretion of urine. If a diuretic is desired, these herbs would be good choices: parsley, watercress, or asparagus leaves or roots. If a diaphoretic is wanted, you could use boneset, yarrow, peppermint, or verbena. A diaphoretic is an agent or sudorific that increases perspiration.

2. *Aromatics:* aromatics have a pleasant smell. Some good examples are mints, fennel, catnip, sassafras bark, and marjoram.

3. *Demulcents:* a demulcent is an agent that soothes or softens. It usually aids the mucous membranes. Here are some examples: mallow, hollyhocks, Irish moss, mullein, slippery elm, honey, and balm of Gilead.

Preparing Tinctures

Learning how to make tinctures means you have another way to use herbs for home treatments. A tincture is nothing more than a highly concentrated liquid extract of herbs. A tincture can be applied externally or taken internally, and they are often made using an alcohol base or an oil base. The oil base needs to have a preservative such as vitamin E or honey added. An oil tincture is most often used externally. An alcohol-based tincture is most frequently used as an internal treatment. If you wish to make a water-based tincture, you can do that too.

The kind of herbs you choose to put in your tinctures depends upon what conditions you need to heal. For example, you would make a tincture of comfrey root to heal and clean sores because comfrey has pain-killing properties and it also aids in cell rejuvenation. If you are choosing herbs to use in a tincture that will be taken orally, be careful to choose "safe" herbs (ones that you know you can safely ingest).

Water-Based Tincture

Fill a glass quart jar half full of the herb(s) chosen and fill with water. Close the lid tightly and place the jar in a small pan filled halfway with water. Slowly bring this water to a boil. Continue boiling for at least 15 minutes. Remove the jar from the water and strain out the herbs. Place the herb water in a sterile container and stir in honey—about half the amount of the herb liquid. I don't like to use standard measurements because I prefer to work with the amount of herbs that I have on hand. After adding the honey as a preservative, it is now a tincture ready for use. Add several droppers of the tincture to tea, juice, or water. Place a few drops under the tongue for immediate benefit.

Alcohol-Based Tincture

To make an alcohol-based tincture, I use vodka, as it has less taste compared to other liquors, but you can use brandy or whatever liquor you wish. Place the herb(s) in a glass quart jar and cover completely with alcohol. Place the closed jar in a warm, sunny area, and let the sun do the work for you. Just leave the jar to steep for about 2 weeks, shaking daily. After 2 weeks, strain out the herbs and place the liquid in a sterile container. The alcohol preserves the tincture, so you don't need to add a preservative. The tincture is now ready for use.

Oil-Based Tincture

An oil-based tincture is made in the same manner as water- and alcohol-based tinctures. Place the herb in a quart jar and cover completely with any oil you would use on your skin. Vegetable, peanut, almond, or olive oil are the most commonly used. Place the jar in a sunny, warm window or other area for 2 weeks. After straining, add honey or vitamin E to the oil as a preservative.

Using Tinctures

There are many ways tinctures can be used, and they can serve many purposes.

Oil-based tinctures can be made into salves by heating them on low heat and adding melted beeswax. Stir until cool and of the consistency desired.

Alcohol-based tinctures can be used many ways. Many people like flavored coffee, and a vanilla-flavored tincture makes a wonderful addition to coffee along with a little cream and sugar. You can enhance the flavor of your cooking by creating your own tinctures with clove, cinnamon, or peppermint. To prepare a vanilla tincture, add 5–6 vanilla beans to 1 pint of alcohol.

Many of the things you buy at the drugstore can be duplicated at home. Even perfumes can be made using the same tincture-making principles. A simple mouthwash exactly like the kinds found at the store can be made by filling a quart jar with water, adding 1 ounce of vodka and several drops of pure peppermint essential oil, and shaking well. Transfer to a pretty jar and label. It is now ready to use. The alcohol preserves the mouthwash and is an astringent too. It is much more economical and safer to prepare your own things. You know what's in them!

Basic Cleansing Cream

The recipe for basic cleansing cream calls for 2 tablespoons beeswax, 4 tablespoons lanolin, 2 tablespoons herbal infusion water (instructions follow), ⅜ cup olive oil, and ⅛ ounce scented oil (if desired). Melt the lanolin and beeswax in a double boiler over low heat. When melted, add the olive oil. Remove from heat and stir in scented oil. Stir continuously until cool. The mixture will thicken and become creamy. Store in a screw-top jar.

Use this cream to clean your face. Apply a small amount and massage into face. Place a hot cloth over face. As the cloth cools, rinse it in hot water to heat it up again. Do this several times.

Remove all traces of cleanser with a clean tissue. Pat some of the herbal infusion on as a skin toner.

Basic Herbal Infusion

To prepare a basic herbal infusion, pour 1½ cups boiling water over the herb of your choice. Use 3–4 tablespoons fresh herb or 1 teaspoon dried herb. Use a chinaware or earthenware container. Steep 30 minutes and strain. Bottle the mixture in a screw-top container and refrigerate. It keeps about a week. Use cold. An infusion has many beneficial effects, depending on the herb used.

chamomile: tones up relaxed muscles.

fennel: an infusion of the leaves and seeds clears up spots.

lemon balm: smooths wrinkles.

mints: all mints are excellent astringents.

rosemary: tightens sagging skin.

comfrey: mix with witch hazel as an excellent tonic to smooth wrinkles.

thyme: an excellent astringent; it helps to clear acne.

Use the infusion at least twice weekly to get best results, though you will probably notice the effects on the first application.

Preparing to Make Soap

One of the first ways you can begin to live a healthy lifestyle is to make your own soap. Many people would like to but think that it is a difficult thing to do. The whole procedure takes about 1½ hours from start to finish. I make soap as I need it and only have to do so a couple of times yearly.

There are no artificial chemicals in this homemade soap and that really is the first step in being chemical free. The ingredients are simple, and there are only a few tools involved. You will need a wooden spoon, a wide-mouthed glass half-gallon jar, several flat containers that you can line with plastic wrap (you could use several shoeboxes if desired), an enamel or iron pot in which to "cook" the soap, molds, and a photography or dairy thermometer. The temperature is important when making soap. Get a good thermometer that registers as low as 95–98 degrees Fahrenheit.

There are several rules to follow when making your soap:

1. Get your containers ready by either greasing them or lining them with plastic wrap. Do this first so that they are ready when needed.

2. Never use aluminum to prepare your soap. Always use enamel, stainless steel, or iron containers. You will use the wide-mouthed glass container to mix your lye solution in, but you will need a container of enamel, stainless steel, or iron to "cook" your soap.

3. Never allow your curing soap to sit in a drafty area, as this will make your finished product hard and flinty. I cover mine with several thicknesses of newspaper and then cover with a folded blanket for several days.

4. Make sure your molds are at least 1½ to 2 inches thick. If the mold is too thin, it will cause the soap to curl. If it is too thick, it will make the soap too big, and it will be difficult to hold.

5. To add scent to your soap, add the scented oil right before you pour the soap into your molds. Any of the scented oils will do. I like to use the vanilla scent for my own personal use, but any that you prefer will do great. Try using a fruity or flower scent. Sometimes kids like the smell of peppermint, and this works great too. You will need to add about 2 tablespoons of the scented oil to each batch. Add more if a stronger scent is desired.

   The scented oils that you add can be of help in treating skin disorders. Lavender oil is an excellent astringent. Adding olive or almond oil is great for dry skin. Thyme oil acts as a deodorant aid. If you prefer, you don't need to add any oils. The plain soap alone is great for your skin because it has no artificial additives in it.

6. When adding the lye to the cold water, please do so slowly and carefully. I never would make soap when the kids were around because I was afraid that they would get into the solution when my back was turned. I have since learned that kittens are very curious, and you need to watch your pets when you make soap. I had a very close call with one of my kittens, so please take certain precautions. Wear rubber gloves and do not breathe in the fumes. The mixture will heat up when you are pouring the lye in the water, so be sure to use very cold water. Stir very slowly to avoid splattering and burning yourself. The splatters will also cause damage to countertops, so you may want to do this procedure outdoors. Making the soap outdoors will also cut down on the fumes.

If you happen to splash any of the solution on your skin, rinse off immediately with water and then rinse the area with vinegar. Vinegar will neutralize the lye somewhat.

Continue stirring until the lye crystals are completely dissolved. You will need to place the jar in a pan (or sink) filled with cold water to bring the temperature of the lye solution back down to 90–95 degrees. After that temperature is reached, slowly add the lye solution to the oil.

Basic Soap Recipe

This recipe is for basic soap. To make your lye solution, add 1½ cups of lye to 5 cups of cold water in your wide-mouth jar. Stir until your lye crystals are completely dissolved. The lye heats the water up. Place the jar in cold water to bring the temperature down to about 90–95 degrees. In an enamel, stainless steel, or iron pan, slowly melt 6 pounds of lard. Place that container in cold water to bring the temperature down to about 120–130 degrees.

When temperatures for both solutions are right, slowly add the lye solution to the melted lard, stirring constantly with a wooden spoon. Keep stirring continuously for about 30 minutes.

Add the scented oil and pour into greased or plastic wrap-lined molds. Cool overnight.

If you use just one container for a mold instead of individual molds, you need to cut the soap into bars the next morning.

Remove the soap from the molds after several days. Age the soap for about 2 weeks before using. Remember that aging only improves your soap.

APPENDIX B

PREPARE YOUR MEDICINE CHEST

As you become more familiar with using different herbal medicines, you will get some idea of which herbs you will need to keep on hand. Also, your family's habits will determine what you keep on hand. It's a personal decision; no one can tell you what you need. If someone in the family has a tendency to get chest colds, you would prepare some of those remedies or at least have on hand different herbs needed to create those remedies so you can treat them at the first sign of illness. Sometimes, by treating a particular illness before it has a chance to get a good hold, we limit the chances of it becoming a serious illness.

By this time, I know what tonics, salves, and tinctures I need for my family. By keeping some of these available, I can be prepared for just about any illness or accident. Here is a list of some of the remedies that I keep on hand. I find that I use some frequently and others hardly at all.

1. Menthol camphorated oil is the first thing I would use on any strained muscle, soreness, or arthritis. It's also my first choice for easing chest tightness. My recipe makes a pint, so this lasts me for some time.

2. I like to keep a good assortment of tinctures on hand. I use a valerian tincture the most. I use it to treat different skin rashes, headaches, and nervousness. If I feel a cold coming on, I use an antibiotic tincture and a rosemary tincture. I usually use calendula to clean cuts and scrapes, but almost any tincture is good for that, so I don't worry too much if I run out of calendula tincture.

3. I always have several salves on hand. I always keep a balm of Gilead salve ready to treat burns and scratches. I have aloe vera growing in several different parts of the house, and I always have the fresh leaves handy, so I am not too concerned with making a salve from that. If I had to tend to a more serious burn, I would make some aloe salve.

4. I keep an earache tincture ready for use. I don't get earaches, but my grandson does, so I keep it for him. I also use it on my dog, Charley, when he is bothered with ear problems. He is eighteen years old now, so I use quite a few of my home remedies to keep him comfortable. He still gets around really well, so the herbs must be of help to him.

5. I always keep wild cherry cough syrup on hand, and in the fall, I try to keep a supply of cough drops. They are delicious. We suck on those even when we don't have a cough.

6. I keep several kinds of herbal capsules prepared for our home use. I take the "change of life" (menopause) capsules, along with the capsules for poor circulation. To save time, and to have them ready when I need them, I try to make at least a two-month supply of the capsules at one time.

7. In the cabinet, I place all the vitamin supplements that we might need to take during bouts of illness. I also stock herbs to make remedies for other, less common needs. The

number of herbs that you keep in stock is not as important as your ability to use what you do have.

The dried herbs found in tea or infusion remedies are effective and easy to use, so just keeping them on hand is enough to enable you to treat many personal illnesses. It may take a little time to get the supplies you need, but it is well worth the effort.

I keep all the cooking herbs in the kitchen spice cabinet. The herbal preparations designed for bath or personal care are kept in the linen closet or bathroom. The personal care products are used daily and, of course, are kept where they will be at hand.

It really doesn't take as much time as you might think to use the herbs and make herbal products for daily use. Even if they did take a lot of time, I still would keep making them for our health's sake.

Besides, I get much pleasure and enjoyment out of being able to make many of the products that are used here in my home. There is a lot of self-satisfaction in using nature's bounty.

SIGNATURES OF HERBS

Many of the herbs have what are called "signatures," a system of characteristics that help identify the herb and its functions. It is important to understand what those signatures are in order to know what the herb can be used for. You will become proficient in gathering wild herbs once you have an understanding of the signatures of the plants. (I want to mention here that with knowledge comes responsibility. Many of the wild herbs are on the endangered list, so be aware when you do use nature's bounty.)

Knowing the signatures of the plants will also help you in preparing and creating your own recipes. Certain characteristics can be broken down into categories. These categories indicate what a particular plant can be used for. Here are some general rules to help you understand signatures.

1. The color of the herb's flowers is an important part of the signature. The plants with yellow blooms are generally used for liver, gallbladder, and all urinary problems and tonics that rid the body of toxins and infections.

The herbs with reddish flowers are all good blood purifiers and/or alteratives. [See glossary for definitions of terms.—Ed.] The color red indicates the astringency or the healing effect of certain herbs. Herbs with this color can be used to treat skin disorders that are caused by blood impurities. The active ingredient of many of the alterative herbs is considered to be antibiotic in nature.

Herbs that have purple or blue flowers are, without exception, used as a sedative or relaxant. These are good to add to a recipe when the patient needs to stay calm during an illness, or in treating muscle spasms. Most of our illnesses are caused by stress, and most herbal remedies would benefit from the addition of a calmative or sedative. They are also considered good blood purifiers, so they have their place as tonics as well.

Always be mindful of the flower colors when gathering herbs for a specific treatment. A good example of differences found in herbs is the sage plant. Sometimes a pink and a blue bloom will be found on the same species of sage growing right next to each other. This would indicate to me that the blue-flowered plant would be used only as a sedative. Because of the astringent nature of sage, both pink- and blue-flowered sage can be used as a blood purifier, but I would choose the pink-blossomed plant because the pink flowers indicate that it has more blood-purifying properties.

The shape of a plant's flowers is also an important characteristic to consider. Many plants, such as eyebright and chamomile, are indicative for eyes because the floral parts resemble eyes.

2. The growing condition of the herb is the second thing you look at to ascertain the signature of the herb. Growing in areas with a lot of gravel indicates that the plants can be used in treating illnesses that have to do with stone or gravel in the body. These herbs help to cleanse and remove harmful accumulations from the alimentary and bronchial systems. They are used to treat kidney stones or gallstones. So-called stone-breakers are parsley, peppergrass, shepherd's purse, sassafras, and mullein. Mullein will grow just about anywhere. I find it quite often growing in gravel along rail-ways and roadways.

  Herbs found growing in mucky, swampy, or wet ground are good to use in recipes designed to treat excessive mucous excretions, such as respiratory problems dealing with asthma, colds, coughs, and rheumatic disorders. Willow, verbena, boneset, and elder are examples of this.

  Herbs that grow near fast-moving water are good to use as diuretics. These help to clean the alimentary systems of toxins and harmful wastes.

3. Different textures indicate different uses. Herbs that have a soft texture to them are useful for treating swollen or inflamed areas. They can also be used for treating so-called wet colds or any chest disorders.

  Horehound, mullein, and hollyhocks are good examples of emollient herbs.

4. Any of the herbs that have thorns or are prickly are used in disorders where there is sharp pain. Thistle is used as a tonic for all the organs. Hawthorn can be used as a tonic for the heart because it has sharp thorns and is indicative of sharp pains in the heart. Hawthorn is also considered a diuretic,

and that is helpful in any heart treatment. Wild prickly lettuce is used as a pain reliever and as a sedative. It has blossoms that may be white, yellow, or blue. The prickles are indicative of its usefulness in treating sharp pain.

The epidermal hairs of some of the plants are suggestive of their use in internal problems where there are sharp or stitching pains. Hops, nettle, and mullein are three plants that come to mind immediately.

5. Any herb that clings to itself is believed to cling to and help remove any hardened mucus of the inner systems. Any of the herbs that have a "sticking to" propensity are good to use in ridding the body of toxins and virus germs. Balm of Gilead is used in chest complaints because it has a sticky substance covering it.

   The ground-covering herbs are also considered good to use in ridding the body of hardened mucus. Examples of these are coltsfoot, sage, thyme, horehound, and mallow.

6. Herbs that are also vines are considered good to use in remedies for the blood system and the nervous system because they resemble them; the blood vessels and the nerve paths throughout the body call to mind the vines.

   Another way to check whether or not the herb will be useful for these disorders is to check the root system of the plant. If it has a veinlike root system, then the herb may be used to treat disorders dealing with the blood system or nervous disorders.

7. The skin healers have several different signatures. They have thin, threadlike roots and stems. Cinquefoil, gold thread, and septfoil are good examples of this. The roots resemble the structure of the veins in the skin.

8. Fissures in the bark of certain trees are indicative of their use in treating certain skin disorders. Cherry, white birch, and elder are examples of trees with healing properties for skin ulcers and sores. Balsamic resinous exudations help to heal cuts and ulcers of the skin.

   Moss and lichens are good choices when making preparations used to treat skin diseases (such as psoriasis) because these herbs resemble the appearance of these disorders.

9. Sometimes, just the name alone can indicate the use of that particular herb. Heartsease, eyebright, pleurisy root, feverfew, cancer root, and throat root are just a few.

10. Many of the herbs that have a root structure resembling the human torso are used as aphrodisiacs or as a way to overcome sterility. Ginseng is an example of this.

    You can find similarities in other ways in the plant world. For example, skullcap was named as such because the flowers resembled helmets, and the walnut resembles the human brain. Such similarities can lead those plants to be used in treatments for headaches and nervous disorders.

11. Another important herbal signature is aroma. Many strong-smelling herbs, such as cinnamon, clove, thyme, and rosemary, are used as disinfectants. Most of the aromatic herbs are highly antiseptic or germicidal and have antibiotic properties. Sage, pennyroyal, all mints, tansy, and yarrow are good examples.

12. Another good rule to remember is that many herbs that attract bees can also be used as an antidote for bee stings and insect bites. Bee balm and basil are good examples of this. Just crush several leaves and rub on the area.

Some of the signatures will not apply in every case. There are some herbs that have no signature. Study the properties of the plant that you plan to use and become familiar with the signatures of that plant (or lack of signatures) before using it in any recipe.

Becoming familiar with the signatures of the herbs is one of the first steps in getting control over our health. When the ancient shamans and healers concentrated on just a few plants and became experts in the use of those few, their remedies were effective. Diet played an important part in their treatments. They realized that a healthy diet was linked to a healthy body and a healthy mind.

We live in a world that has become dangerous to our health, and we should start where we can do the most good. Taking care of those we love and teaching them to take care of their body, spirit, and mind is the most important difference we can make. By studying the ways Mother Nature can make our life better, we also become more spiritually minded. We soon realize that we are all connected and learn ways to deal with our own excesses. We learn to work with nature and not against it. We learn that we are responsible for our own health and take steps to stay healthy.

HERB PROPERTIES

Astringents

Astringents are natural cleansers and are antibiotic in nature.

balm of Gilead

bee balm

borage

calendula

chervil

cinnamon

comfrey

eyebright

garlic

hyssop

lemon balm

mints (all)

mullein

nettle

plantain

rosemary

sage

shepherd's purse

sweet basil

tansy

thyme

white yarrow

willow bark

witch hazel

Diuretics

Diuretics increase the output of urine, taking harmful substances from the system.

apple

asparagus

balm of Gilead

borage

burdock

carrot

chamomile

chervil

comfrey

corn silk

cramp bark

dandelion

elder

garden strawberry

heartsease

lemon balm

mugwort

mullein

nasturtium

nettle

parsley

pennyroyal

plantain

red raspberry

sage

savory

shepherd's purse

St. John's wort

sweet basil

thyme

watercress

wild strawberry

Expectorants

These herbs cause the expulsion of mucus and break up congestion.

anise

balm of Gilead

basil

bee balm

betony

blue cohosh

boneset

borage

catnip

chamomile

chervil

chicory

coltsfoot

comfrey

corn flowers

costmary

cramp bark

elecampane root

garlic

ginger

heartsease

hollyhocks

hops

horehound

horseradish

hyssop

Irish moss

lavender

lemon balm

lemon verbena

lettuce

lobelia

marshmallow

motherwort

mullein

nettle

prickly lettuce

sassafras

slippery elm

St. John's wort

sweet cicely

wild cherry bark

Nervines

Nervines relieve nervous irritation caused by strain and tension.

basil

borage

blue cohosh

catnip

chamomile

chervil

chicory

comfrey

corn flower

cramp bark

heartsease

hops

lavender

lettuce

lobelia

motherwort

nettle

passionflower

pennyroyal

prickly lettuce

red clover

rosemary

sage

sassafras

skullcap

slippery elm

St. John's wort

sweet cicely

valerian

violet

wild cherry bark

willow

yarrow

Stimulants

These herbs increase stimuli to the system and will increase blood circulation.

anise

balm of Gilead

blue cohosh

calendula

caraway seed

cayenne pepper

chervil

cinnamon

cloves

coriander seed

ginger root

ginseng

hyssop

lemon balm

lobelia

mints (all)

nettle

parsley

pennyroyal

raspberry

red clover

rosemary

sage

shepherd's purse

St. John's wort

valerian

white yarrow

yerba santa

Tonics

Tonics benefit the whole body. They strengthen the organs that are affected by the action of the digestive system. They do take time to work, so keep the treatment going until the system has time to adjust.

anise

burdock

cayenne pepper

chicory

cinnamon

comfrey

corn silk

costmary

dandelion

ginger

ginseng

heartsease

hops

lavender

lemon balm

mints (all)

mullein

nasturtium

nettle

parsley

red clover

red raspberry

rosemary

sassafras

shepherd's purse

violet

white yarrow

willow bark

WHICH PART OF THE HERB IS USED?

I have listed a few of the herbs that would be used in making some of the recipes. I've also included information on which part of the herb is commonly used to prepare remedies.

Acacia (*Acacia senegal*)
The exudation is the part used. Removes phlegm from the throat and bronchia. Used for conditions of the respiratory and digestive organs.

Alkanet (*Alkanna tinctoria*)
The root is the part used. Used for blood disorders and liver and gall-bladder problems.

Allspice (*Lindera benzoin*)
Fruit, leaves, and twigs are used. Breaks fevers.

Angelica (*Angelica archangelica*)
Roots, seeds, and leaves are used. Expectorant for colds and coughs. Also treats kidney disorders and aids the digestive system.
    Caution: Be careful not to mistake poison hemlock for angelica.

Anise (*Pimpinella anisum*)

The leaves and seeds are used. Anise is good for colds and flu. Licorice or anise hyssop is a great tea to relieve fever. It is used as a digestive aid. It can be added to recipes for teas that include unpleasant-tasting herbs. Anise adds a nice licorice flavor to any tea.

Apple (*Pyrus malus*)

The whole fruit is used. Dried apple tea is an excellent diuretic. Aids in elimination of toxins from the system.

Asparagus (*Asparagus officinalis*)

The shoots and the roots are used. Warm tea made from asparagus is used as an excellent diuretic. Drink every 2–3 hours.

Balm of Gilead (*Populus candicans*)

The closed bud of the poplar tree is the part used. It is an expectorant for chest ailments and bronchial disorders.

Basil (*Ocimum basilicum*)

The leaves are used. Basil aids in digestion and is used as a mild laxative. Since it also acts as a mild sedative, it is used to treat headaches.
Caution: Can cause allergies and skin irritation.

Bee Balm (*Monarda didyma*)

All of the plant can be used. Bee balm is used as an antiseptic because it contains thymol and removes impurities from the blood. Also used to stimulate the liver and spleen.

Black Alder (*Prinos verticillatus*)

Bark and fruits are used. Good treatment for liver and gallbladder problems. Cleans the system of accumulated mucoid toxins.

Blackberry (*Rubus* spp.)

Leaves, fruit, and roots are used for different illnesses. Dissolves deposits in the alimentary system as well as the kidneys.

Boneset (*Eupatorium perfoliatum*)

The upper half of the herb is used. Has a cleansing effect on all the organs. Used as a tonic as well as an aid in eliminating mucus from the alimentary, bronchial, bowel, and liver systems.

Also a muscle relaxant.

Borage (*Borago officinalis*)

Leaves and flowers are used. Borage has a cucumber taste and makes a cooling addition to teas. Borage is often used to help relieve depression. The flowers, made into a tea, are used to treat fevers and colds.

Calendula (*Calendula officinalis*)

The flowers are used in remedies for many different illnesses. The tea is used internally and externally. It has been used to stop bleeding and has antibiotic properties to heal wounds. Use for chest ailments as well as for cramps, flu, and stomach problems, and as an aid to induce sweating to bring down fever.

Catnip (*Nepeta cataria*)

Leaves and flowering tops are used to treat colic or flatulence.

Celery (*Apium graveolens*)

Tea made from celery cases the stomach and is used as a nervine and sedative. Always use fresh celery. Never use celery that is limp or discolored, even to cook with.

Chamomile (*Anthemis nobilis, Matricaria chamomilla*)

Flowers and the upper half of the plant are used. It is a calmative and sedative. Treats headaches and cramps and other gastrointestinal disorders.

Chicory (*Cichorium intybus*)

The flowers are used as a sedative and general tonic. It is also used as a diuretic.

Clary Sage (*Salvia sclarea*)

The leaves and seeds are used. Not only is clary sage used for eye disorders, but it has great properties that help to clear the sediments from the liver and kidneys. The tea is also used to help with stomach and intestinal problems. Good for nausea and colic treatment.

Cleavers (*Galium aparine*)

The entire herb is useful. A strong diuretic, it is used to dissolve deposits in the kidneys.

Coltsfoot (*Tussilago farfara*)

The leaves are the part used. This herb binds to toxins in the system and helps to eliminate them. Great expectorant.

Caution: Coltsfoot should be avoided if you have liver issues.

Corn silk (*Zea mays*)

Corn silk is a great diuretic. Use to clean the urinary system and as a tonic for the whole system. Dry plenty of it so that you can use it during the winter months for kidney and bladder infections.

Dandelion (*Taraxacum officinale*)
Roots and leaves are used. Use as a general tonic, as well as for liver and gallbladder complaints.

Elder (*Sambucus canadensis*)
Leaves, fruits, and flowers are used. Elder flower tea is an excellent diuretic. Use for feverish colds too.

Eyebright (*Euphrasia officinalis*)
Use the seeds if you have a tendency toward kidney stones. Use in a rinse for eyes.

Fennel (*Foeniculum vulgare*)
All parts are used. Aids digestion and helps calm nervous stomach. Increases milk production.

Fenugreek (*Trigonella foenum-graecum*)
Use the seeds. Soothes the lining of the stomach and intestines.

Ginseng (*Panax quinquefolius*)
The root is used. For centuries it has been considered a near cure-all. Used as a tonic for all the systems of the body and as an aphrodisiac.

Hollyhock (*Alcea rosea*)
Roots and leaves are used. Leaves can be used uncooked in salads or cooked as a side dish. It is an emollient and good to use during colds. Use if prone to kidney stones.

Horehound (*Marrubium vulgare*)
Flowering tops and leaves are used. Use for bronchial and stomach disorders. Good for sore throats and colds. It is an expectorant.

Irish Moss (*Chondrus crispus, Gigartina mamillosa*)
The dried plant is used. Use in bronchial disorders and for kidney problems. Use in cough syrups.

Kelp (*Fucus vesiculosus*)
Kelp contains iodine. Use to purify the blood as well as for goiters.

Kidney Beans (*Phaseolus vulgaris*)
Tea made from the beans and pods is considered to be of a diuretic nature. It helps to clean the kidneys and ureters of gravel.

Lavender (*Lavandula angustifolia*)
The flowers make a pleasant tea that has sedative properties. Use for releasing tension and headaches.

Lemon Balm (*Melissa officinalis*)
The leaves make a tea with a sedative action. Use to induce sweating to reduce fevers. It also regulates menstruation.

Lemon Verbena (*Aloysia triphylla*)
The leaves make a tea for upset stomachs; also has a tonic effect upon the intestines. It has a slight sedative effect and can be used to relax as well as reduce the fever of colds and flu.

Licorice (*Glycyrrhiza glabra*)

The root is the part used. Has estrogen-like properties, so use during and after change of life. Use also for all blood and bronchial problems.

Caution: Do not use if you have heart issues or high blood pressure.

Marsh Mallow (*Althaea officinalis*)

The root is used to soothe inflammations and irritations of the urinary and alimentary systems. Will help to dispel hoarseness and tickling of the throat, as well as help in all bronchial disorders.

Mullein (*Verbascum thapsus*)

The flowers and leaves are the parts most used, but every part can be used. Used for bronchial problems, as well as to inhibit the growth of certain bacteria. It is great to use during colds, as it has antibiotic properties.

Nettle (*Urtica dioica*)

The leaves and upper part of the plant are used. Used to help relieve arthritis pains. Also frequently used in remedies for losing weight.

Nutmeg (*Myristica fragrans*)

Use in small doses to help stomach disorders and digestion.

Caution: It is a powerful narcotic if used in too large a dose.

Pansy (*Viola tricolor*)

The whole herb is used. A mild expectorant. Used for colds and asthma. Good tonic for the heart. Pansy is also known as heartsease.

Parsley (*Petroselinum crispum*)
The whole herb is used. Great diuretic. Parsley tea has long been used to treat kidney problems.

Pennyroyal (*Mentha pulegium*)
The leaves of the herb are used, most often in remedies combined with other herbs. Relieves upset stomach and is a gentle stimulant. Good to use for menstrual cramps because it stimulates the uterine muscles.

Peppermint (*Mentha piperita*)
Leaves and the flowering tops are the parts used. Removes hardened mucus from the alimentary and bronchial systems. Used for discomfort of colds and stomach problems.

Plantain (*Plantago major*)
Roots and leaves are used. Plantain has antiseptic properties and removes toxins from the system.

Pokeweed (*Phytolacca americana*)
The early shoots are used, as are the roots and berries. Pokeweed should be used with caution in any home remedy. I call it the chemotherapy of the herbs, as it is an extremely strong purge. It duplicates the effects of cortisone, which stimulates the entire glandular system. It is used only when drastic measures are called for and when all other natural methods have failed or are not suitable. It serves as an incredibly powerful laxative and diuretic to clean the whole system.

Caution: Use with care. Please keep children away from the berries. They are fascinated by the beautiful berries, but it is not a safe plant for children to be around.

Prickly Lettuce (*Lactuca virosa, L. serriola*)

The leaves and gum are used. Use as a strong sedative to treat insomnia. Also removes hardened excretions from the bronchial system.

Purslane (*Portulaca oleracea*)

The herb above the ground is the part used. It is a good diuretic and cleanser for the kidneys. I have given it to goats that were suffering from scours (diarrhea). I made a tea with the purslane and then forced it down their throats. It saved some of my goats from death.

Raspberry (*Rubus idaeus*)

The leaves and fruit are used. Raspberry leaf tea stimulates the kidneys. The main purpose of the tea is to relax the uterine muscles. The roots are well known for their astringent properties. Because the root has concentrations of tannic and gallic acids, it has antibiotic value.

Red Clover (*Trifolium pratense*)

The flowering tops are used. Great blood purifier and tonic. Most skin disorders are caused by impurities of the blood, and this tea should be taken on a regular basis if you suffer from pimples, boils, or other skin eruptions.

Caution: Some people are allergic to red clover.

Rose Hips (*Rosa canina*)

The hips, leaves, and flowers are used. Great tonic for the blood. The hips contain vitamin P, which prevents and heals ruptures of small blood vessels. Treatment of the kidneys is indicated by the citric acids in the hips.

Rosemary (*Rosmarinus officinalis*)

The needles are used as an astringent. It does relax the muscles and is used to treat depression, muscle spasms, and headaches.

Sage (*Salvia officinalis*)

The leaves are used. Sage is a stimulating herb for the kidneys and helps to remove toxins from the system. The sedative properties are well known, so it can be used to treat headaches. Also used to treat colds because it removes catarrh in the alimentary and bronchial systems.

Caution: Sage can cause symptoms of poisoning if taken in excess. Also, do not use if pregnant or breastfeeding; it can cause the mammary glands to dry up.

Sassafras (*Sassafras albidum*)

The bark of the root is most commonly used to break up impurities in the blood system, so it is considered a blood purifier and thinner. It has a gentle cleansing action that is helpful to the kidneys.

Sheep's Sorrel (*Rumex acetosella*)

The plant above ground is used. Great to reduce fevers. It is used for blood disorders and cleans the urinary system. The word *sorrel* means sour. It is called sorrel for the acidity in the leaves.

Shepherd's Purse (*Capsella bursa-pastoris*)

The entire plant is used. It has a stimulating effect upon the uterine muscles. Also used in cases of diarrhea for humans and animals because of the astringent properties. It has hemostatic properties (stops bleeding), so it is useful for all kinds of hemorrhages affecting the uterus, lungs, stomach, and kidneys. Shepherd's purse also increases the flow of urine and is helpful in removing mucous matter from the urine.

Skullcap (*Scutellaria lateriflora*)

The part above ground is used. The sedative properties are well known. Used for insomnia, nervous disorders, and headaches.

Slippery Elm (*Ulmus rubra*)

The dried inner bark is the part used. A mild expectorant, it soothes irritations of the alimentary and bronchial systems.

Solomon's Seal (*Polygonatum officinale*)

The root is the part used as a diuretic, and it also has mucilaginous properties that help with vigorous expectoration during bronchial disorders.

Spearmint (*Mentha spicata*)

Leaves and flowering tops are used. Great for treating colic and disturbances of the alimentary system. Used as a diuretic also.

Sweet Woodruff (*Galium odoratum*)

The top part of the herb is used. Sweet woodruff has a very pleasant smell after it starts to dry. It has been used as a blood purifier and as a tonic for the heart and the liver. It is also used as a calmative, helping to soothe stomach disorders and upsets.

Tag Alder (*Alnus serrulata*)

Cones and bark are used as a diuretic.

Thyme (*Thymus vulgaris*)

The whole top of the growing herb is used. Has a therapeutic action on the bronchial system. It is a stimulant and has antiseptic properties for use in cleaning the alimentary, urinary, and bronchial systems.

Valerian (*Valeriana officinalis*)

The root is the part used. Valerian has a very unpleasant smell, but its influence on the brain and spinal cord are well known. It acts like valium but without the side effects of addiction that you would have with the prescription drug. It is a great calmative and is used extensively for sleeplessness and nervous disorders.

Caution: Do not use if you have stomach or heart issues.

Vervain (*Verbena hastata*)

The entire herb is used. The plant has diaphoretic and expectorant properties, so is great to use for chest complaints like feverish colds or pleurisy.

Violet (*Viola odorata*)

The flowers, leaves, and roots are used. Violets contain more vitamin A than any other known plant. It's a great tonic and is a mild sedative too. The roots of violets are known to soothe stomach pains and stop diarrhea.

Watercress (*Nasturtium officinale*)

The entire plant is used. Cleans the kidneys and is loaded with vitamin C. Contains many important minerals, such as calcium, sulfur, copper, iron, and manganese, which strengthen the blood. It's a great tea to treat anemic conditions as well as being a great all-around tonic.

Caution: Do not use if pregnant or breastfeeding.

Wild Ginger (*Asarum canadense*)

The root is the part used. Wild ginger is a stimulant and diuretic. The herb acts on the kidneys to eliminate viscous matter. Also a great tonic for the whole body.

Wild Strawberry (*Fragaria virginiana*) and Garden Strawberry (*Fragaria vesca*)

The roots, leaves, and berries are used. Drinking a tea made from strawberry leaves is a quick way to add minerals to the blood system. There is iron, potassium, sulfur, calcium, sodium, and the associated acids, such as citric and malic, in the herb. The fruit contains vitamin C, so it is useful to treat scurvy. It is used to treat gout and related disorders. Has great benefits for the alimentary and urinary system. An all-around fantastic tonic.

Wild Yam (*Dioscorea villosa*)

The root is used. Wild yam is treated by the body as though it is estrogen and so is of great help during menopausal stages. Used in the treatment of asthma and other ailments affecting the bronchial system.

Willow (*Salix* spp.)

The twigs, leaves, and bark are used. Contains salicin and salicylates—source of the first aspirin. Good to take for headaches, aches, and pains of arthritic conditions and to help relieve pain during menstruation. Good to use alone or mixed with other herbs to relieve discomfort of colds and flu.

Woad (*Genista tinctoria*)

The entire plant has a use. Not only does it supply us with the only natural blue dye (through use of the root), but the leaves supply us with a remedy for treating obstructions in the gall bladder and liver.

Yarrow (*Achillea millefolium*)

The whole herb is used. Great to use for feverish ailments. Contains salicin and salicylates, so it eases feverish aches and pains. Combine with more pleasant-tasting herbs to make a tea. The roots are used to treat blood disorders. Yarrow has many minerals in it, such as iron, calcium, potassium, sodium, and sulfur. It also contains two substances called achillein and achilleic acid. When ingested, these substances help to reduce the time that it takes for blood to clot. It has external uses as well. It is an astringent and can be used to clean—as well as relieve the pain of—wounds and sores.

GLOSSARY

acne: an inflammatory disease of the sebaceous glands and hair follicles of the skin.

alimentary canal or tract: the digestive tube from the mouth to the anus, including the mouth, pharynx, esophagus, stomach, large and small intestines, and rectum.

alterative: helps to alter or correct minor functional disorders of the system. Also called a blood purifier.

anemia: a condition in which the blood is deficient in red blood cells or in hemoglobin.

antibiotic: natural substance that inhibits growth or destroys microorganisms. Used to treat infectious diseases.

antiseptic: substance that checks the growth or action of microorganisms.

aphrodisiac: excites sexual desire.

aromatic: has an agreeable odor and slightly stimulative action or properties.

arthritis: inflammation of a joint, accompanied by pain and swelling.

astringent: an agent that has a binding or constricting effect, as when it checks hemorrhages or secretions by coagulation of proteins on a cell surface.

blood purifier: see *alterative.*

bronchitis: inflammation of the mucous membrane of the bronchial system.

catarrh: simple inflammation of the mucous membrane in the respiratory tract.

colic: cramping of the stomach or intestines.

decoction: the liquid left after boiling the herb root or bark to extract the properties.

demulcent: soothing properties in specific herbs that allay the action of stimulating or overactive herbs. Soothing to irritated mucous membranes.

diaphoretic: increases perspiration. Aids in removing toxins and wastes through the skin.

diuretic: increases the flow of urine and aids in elimination of waste products and toxins through the urine.

eczema: acute or chronic inflammatory condition of the skin. May manifest as crusts, scales, or pustules—alone or in combination. More of a symptom than a disease.

emollient: use externally and internally for a soothing or healing effect.

epidermal: outer layer of skin.

excretions: waste matter. The elimination of waste products from the body.

expectorant: facilitates the expulsion of mucus from the respiratory tract.

exudation: oozing of fluids or accumulation of fluid in a cavity.

flatulence: excessive gas in the alimentary canal.

germicidal: any agent that destroys germs or microorganisms.

gravel: the formation of small concretions in the urinary passages.

infusion: the process of steeping herbs in boiling or hot water to extract the properties of the herb. Used as a tea.

laxative: corrects constipation by increasing bowel movements.

mucilaginous: gummy or sticky substance that is soothing to areas that are inflamed.

mucous membrane: membrane lining passages and cavities communicating with the air.

mucus: a protective lubricant coating by cells and glands of the mucous membranes.

nervine: treatment for the nervous system. Quiets nervous irritation due to excitement, fatigue, grief, or headaches.

pleurisy: Inflammation of the membranes that envelope the lungs and thorax.

poultice: herbs that are finely ground and then moistened and applied to an affected area.

psoriasis: chronic, genetically determined lesions of the skin.

relaxant: substance that relieves stress, strain, and tension.

rheumatism: painful inflammation and swelling of muscles and joints.

sedative: soothes nervous excitement and has a quieting effect upon the nervous system without having a narcotic effect.

spasm: involuntary contraction of a muscle or a muscle fiber.

steep: to extract the essence of an herb by soaking it in liquid.

stimulant: increases functional actions of the body; also called an activator.

tonic: restores strength to the whole system and helps different organs.

uterine: relates to the uterus or the womb.

BIBLIOGRAPHY

Calver, Leonie A., Barrie J. Stokes, and Geoffrey K. Isbister. "The Dark Side of the Moon." *The Medical Journal of Australia* 191, no. 11 (August 2009): 692–94.

Carter, Mary Ellen, and William A. McGarey. *Edgar Cayce on Healing*. Edited by Hugh Lynn Cayce. New York: Warner Books, 1971.

Jarvis, D. C. *Folk Medicine: A New England Almanac of Natural Health Care from a Noted Vermont Country Doctor*. New York: Random House Publishing Group, 1995.

Kukuk, Emma. "Under the Spell of the Seasons: Navigating Mental Health in Nature." *Gather Round* (blog). Department of Natural Resources, September 226, 2020.

Weed, Susun S. *Healing Wise*. Wise Woman Herbal. Woodstock, NY: Ash Tree Publishing, 1989.

Xu, Alison Jing, and Aparna A. Labroo. "Incandescent Affect," *Journal of Consumer Psychology* 24, no. 2 (April 2014): 207–216. https://www.jstor.org/stable/26617996.

To Write to the Author

If you wish to contact the author or would like more information about this book, please write to the author in care of Llewellyn Worldwide Ltd. and we will forward your request. Both the author and the publisher appreciate hearing from you and learning of your enjoyment of this book and how it has helped you. Llewellyn Worldwide Ltd. cannot guarantee that every letter written to the author can be answered, but all will be forwarded. Please write to:

Carly Wall
℅ Llewellyn Worldwide
2143 Wooddale Drive
Woodbury, MN 55125-2989

Please enclose a self-addressed stamped envelope for reply, or $1.00 to cover costs. If outside the U.S.A., enclose an international postal reply coupon.

Many of Llewellyn's authors have websites with additional information and resources. For more information, please visit our website at http://www.llewellyn.com.